T0291002

A Parent's Guide to **Tics** and **Tourette's Disorder**

A Parent's Guide to
Tics and
Tourette's
Disorder

NIGEL S. BAMFORD, MD

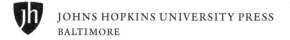 JOHNS HOPKINS UNIVERSITY PRESS
BALTIMORE

Note to the Reader: This book is not meant to substitute for medical care, and treatment should not be based solely on its contents. This book is meant to facilitate dialogue between families and physicians.

Drug dosage: The author and publisher have made reasonable efforts to determine that the selection of drugs discussed in this text conforms to the practices of the general medical community. In view of ongoing research, changes in governmental regulation, and the constant flow of information relating to drug therapy and drug reactions, the reader is urged to check the package insert of each drug for any change in indications and dosage and for warnings and precautions. This is particularly important when the recommended agent is a new and/or infrequently used drug.

© 2025 Johns Hopkins University Press
All rights reserved. Published 2025
Printed in the United States of America on acid-free paper
9 8 7 6 5 4 3 2 1

Johns Hopkins University Press
2715 North Charles Street
Baltimore, Maryland 21218
www.press.jhu.edu

Library of Congress Cataloging-in-Publication Data

Names: Bamford, Nigel S., author.
Title: A parent's guide to tics and Tourette's disorder / Nigel S. Bamford, MD.
Description: Baltimore : Johns Hopkins University Press, 2025. | Series: A Johns Hopkins Press health book | Includes bibliographical references and index.
Identifiers: LCCN 2024021302 | ISBN 9781421449548 (hardcover) | ISBN 9781421449555 (paperback) | ISBN 9781421449562 (epub)
Subjects: LCSH: Tourette syndrome in children—Popular works. | Tic disorders—Popular works.
Classification: LCC RJ496.T68 B36 2025 | DDC 616.8/3—dc23/eng/20240524
LC record available at https://lccn.loc.gov/2024021302

A catalog record for this book is available from the British Library.

Special discounts are available for bulk purchases of this book. For more information, please contact Special Sales at specialsales@jh.edu.

Contents

Preface

Tics are abrupt movements and vocalizations frequently seen in elementary school–aged children. Tics are very common and often short-lived but frightening to parents. Occasionally, tics will persist and interfere with the child's activities. While the internet contains abundant information about tic disorders, much of it is too tightly focused, confusing, or, sometimes, simply inaccurate.

This guide is intended to answer almost all the questions a parent, caregiver, patient, pediatrician, teacher, or health care provider might have about the diagnosis and treatment of tics and Tourette's disorder. The guide also discusses other co-occurring conditions and provides an introduction to brain pathways and mechanisms that may cause tics. The reader will be left with a better understanding of medical terminology that will help them navigate the health care system while they seek answers and relief from tics.

The information provided in this guide is for general informational purposes only and is not intended to be a substitute for professional medical advice, diagnosis, or treatment. Always seek the advice of your health care provider with any questions regarding a medical condition. Never disregard professional medical advice or delay seeking medical advice because of information contained in this guide.

The reader looking for specific advice should seek a professional who is licensed and knowledgeable in the subject. The citations are included in good faith, and the author cannot guarantee the validity of the referenced materials. A glossary of terms used in this guide is provided following the appendix. The word "parent" is meant to include guardians and caregivers. The patient stories included here describe typical presentations and outcomes for children seen in the author's movement disorders clinic. Their similarity to any one particular patient is coincidental.

Acknowledgments

I want to thank my wife, Lisa, my son, Ian, and all of the patients who come to see me to evaluate and treat their movement disorders. I would also like to thank Kathryn McVicar, MD, Kim Levinson, APRN, and Alejandra Madlener, MPH, LCSW, at Yale New Haven Hospital for their critical reviews of the manuscript. Science from the Bamford Laboratory cited in this book was supported by the National Institute of Neurological Disorders and Stroke of the National Institutes of Health under award R01NS060803.

A Parent's Guide to **Tics** and **Tourette's Disorder**

CHAPTER 1

Defining
Tics and
Tourette's
Disorder

A tic is a spontaneous motor movement, a simple vocalization, or a short word. The tic is generated in response to a preceding sensation called a premonitory urge. The tic partially and temporarily relieves the urge, like an itch that is momentarily reduced by scratching.

Tics typically have an onset between the ages of 4 and 6 years.[1] Many children will have short-lived tics that quickly disappear. Other children will develop persistent tics that tend to peak in severity by 10–12 years old. Tics wax and wane over time and change in character and location. By early adulthood, approximately 75 percent of those who experienced tics will have greatly diminished symptoms, and more than one-third will be tic-free.[1] Some children, however, will grow up to have long-lasting motor and vocal tics, and these persons may be diagnosed with Tourette's disorder. Another name for Tourette's disorder is Tourette's syndrome.

What Are Motor and Vocal Tics?

Motor tics are short, abrupt, nonrhythmic, and self-similar movements generally confined to the upper body, including the face, head, neck, and shoulders. These simple movements are similar to those that might be seen in newborns. Simple motor tics can accompany more complex motor movements involving other body parts. Complex motor tics may include repetitive hand opening and closing, skipping, jumping, odd breathing patterns, and the like. Complex movements of the limbs may take the form of obsessive-compulsive behaviors, especially when the limb movements are counted or occur in a series of twos or threes. Complex motor tics that involve rude and inappropriate gestures, called copropraxia, are uncommon. Unlike most other movements, tics can occur automatically. While the tics can be striking to the observer, they are often unnoticeable to the person who has them.

Vocal tics may occur in the presence or absence of motor tics. A simple verbal tic is sometimes called a phonic tic. It is an unintelligible noise that occurs when breathing is combined with the movement of the vocal cords. Examples of vocal tics include a gasp, sniff, grunt, squeak, or other simple sounds. Similar to motor tics, vocal tics may also become more complex. The noises can join together to form patterns or words. On rare occasions, complex vocal tics may consist of offensive four-letter words, referred to as coprolalia. Like motor tics, the sounds and words are abrupt, loud, short, striking, and predictable in character but not in occurrence. They may be unnoticed by the person with tics, especially when the person is very young.

A person with tics may mimic or echo the mouth movements (echomimia), words (echolalia), or actions (echopraxia) of those with whom they are speaking. This mimicry of movements or sounds occurs in up to 20 percent of those with persistent motor and vocal tics.[2] Both echomimia and echolalia can happen without other vocal or motor tics. They can be found in many people who don't have tics, as well as those with autism spectrum disorder and other neuropsychological disorders. While the imitation of movements, behaviors, and sounds is part of childhood development, echomimia and echolalia can become problematic when repetitive.

Unlike most other movement disorders where the subject is aware of the movement, tics can be largely unrecognized by the person with a tic disorder. Young children, in particular, are often unaware of their tics. Unfortunately, a parent or another observer may become annoyed, convinced that such movements and sounds are meant to create disruption and receive attention. Therefore, it is not unusual for a parent, sibling, friend, or teacher to criticize someone with tics because they do not understand the involuntary nature of the movement or sound. This leads to a stressful environment that can increase the frequency and severity of the tic. Fortunately, these issues are often temporary and stop after a diagnosis of a tic disorder is made and the family learns more about it.

Provisional tic disorder

A mother brought her 6-year-old boy to a physician for strange movements. For the past three weeks, she had seen him moving his right shoulder toward the side of his face. The movements mainly occurred when he was watching videos or playing with his digital tablet. When the mother asked the boy what he was doing, he looked puzzled, and the movements stopped for a short time. The parents made no further mention of the movements, and they stopped four weeks later.

Most children who develop tics will have mild and transient tics that are unnoticed by others, including their parents. For those who continue to manifest motor tics or develop vocal tics, parents may seek a clinician's opinion. Generally, two groups of people receive a medical evaluation. The first group consists of young children who are brought to a clinician by a parent. The parent is concerned and perhaps alarmed, but the child is unaware of the problem. The second group consists of older children with painful or uncomfortable tics or adolescents whose persistent tics negatively affect their schoolwork and social activities. They may request help from their parents, who arrange a clinic visit in the hope of finding some relief. While a cure is not available and treatments are imperfect, education about the tic disorder, combined with a determined effort at using psychological and medical interventions, can often bring these older children a degree of relief and improved well-being.

Who Was Georges Gilles de la Tourette?

A tic disorder is sometimes referred to as Tourette's disorder or Tourette's syndrome. Parents often wonder whether a child with tics has Tourette's disorder. Is Tourette's disorder serious? Are any special tests needed to diagnose it? Will a diagnosis of Tourette's disorder help the parent obtain services or tailored treatments for their child? Will the child with a diagnosis of Tourette's disorder have lifelong tics? Briefly reviewing the history of Georges Gilles de la Tourette may shed light on these questions. The disorder he described more than 100 years ago is not the same disorder that we now call Tourette's disorder or syndrome. Gilles de la Tourette believed that it was a lifelong and devastating condition. This is certainly not the case.

Tic disorder was first recorded centuries before Gilles de la Tourette by the ancient Greeks. Commonly referred to as *maladie des tics*, the disorder was described in detail by Georges Albert Édouard Brutus Gilles de la Tourette in 1885. Gilles de la Tourette (1857–1904), like other early pioneers in clinical psychology and psychiatry, including Sigmund Freud, had been a student of Professor Jean-Martin Charcot (1825–1893).[3] Charcot worked and taught at Pitié-Salpêtrière Hospital in Paris, France, and drew students and patients from all over Europe. Charcot was perhaps the world's first neurologist and neuropsychologist who sought to understand the brain's inner workings. His interests spanned many medical disciplines, but he is best known for his work on hysteria, an exaggerated or uncontrollable emotion or excitement he thought may occur in people predisposed to it. At the time, the fame of a great physician was proportionate to the number of students who followed the professor from one patient to the next. These students, including Gilles de la Tourette, often helped to describe the clinical features of a disease and patients' responses to various treatments.

Charcot's mentorship of Gilles de la Tourette—as well as his having a great source of patients with severe maladie des tics—culminated in the well-received published description of the disorder in 1885.[4] In the two-part article, Gilles de la Tourette described the case histories of nine patients who manifested multiple motor tics and involuntary vocalizations that eventually erupted into cursing, which he called "coprolalia."[5] He called the new disease *maladie des tics convulsifs avec coprolalie*, which translates to "convulsive tic disease with coprolalia." At the time, maladie des tics was thought to be a form of chorea. The movements seen in chorea are characterized by brief, irregular muscle contractions that are not repetitive or rhythmic and that appear to flow from one muscle or limb to the next. Gilles de la Tourette showed that convulsive tic disease with coprolalia was, however, a different disorder. Convulsive tic disease with coprolalia also differed from hysteria, an emotional behavior that seems excessive and out of control. He noted that its symptoms might wax and wane, and the disease ultimately resisted all treatments. He thought its outcome to be poor, with no hope of a complete cure; he noted that "once a ticcer, always a ticcer."[6,7] We now know that this is not true for most patients.

Gilles de la Tourette and Charcot argued that they had discovered a new disease. The disease had a definitive set of signs and symptoms, would last lifelong, had a hereditary cause, and would worsen as it passed down generations of an affected family.[7,8] This characterization of convulsive tic disease was challenged, however, by others who noted that tics, coprolalia, and echolalia were found both in patients with maladie des tics and in those with chorea or hysteria.[9] Therefore, it was decided that Tourette's disease could be properly diagnosed only when symptoms persisted and the patient resisted all intervention and had a proven family history of worsening tics.[9]

Over the past century, it has become clear that those diagnosed by Gilles de la Tourette were outliers: they were few in number and showed the more severe symptoms of a tic disorder. Furthermore, tics are better described as a disorder than a disease because the symptoms have no identifiable cause. Thus, the convulsive tic disease of Gilles de la Tourette is not the same as what is called Tourette's disorder or syndrome today. As discussed in the following sections, a diagnosis of Tourette's disorder depends on the type of tic and the duration of symptoms. Furthermore, although our knowledge of genetics has dramatically expanded, and it is believed that the disorder may be passed through some families, the severity of the disorder does not necessarily worsen with successive generations.

What Is Our Current Understanding of Tics and Tourette's Disorder?

While Gilles de la Tourette and Charcot changed how society reacted to people with a tic disorder, it largely remained a psychological disorder with various suspected causes. Until the 1960s, there was little interest in studying the neurological cause of a tic disorder. This changed with the introduction of antipsychotic medications developed and used to treat mental diseases such as schizophrenia. One of these medications, haloperidol, was quite effective in treating people with psychosis; it was also found to be quite effective in treating people with tics. These antipsychotic medications were found to prevent the binding of chemical messengers, called neurotransmitters, to their receptors in the brain. These discoveries were not consistent with the psychological explanations that had been proposed to cause tics. Instead, physicians and scientists began wondering whether tics were caused by subtle changes in the connections that exist between brain cells. Could alterations in brain chemistry or brain structure produce tics? Better treatments can be developed if one understands how a disorder occurs.

Over the past 60 years, many anatomical and physiological experiments have been performed. Sophisticated brain imaging tests, electrical studies called electroencephalograms (or EEGs), antibody testing, pathological studies, and genetic evaluations of affected families have all been performed.[10] While research has excluded fundamental conditions such as brain tumors, stroke, and epilepsy, it has not yet explained the specific brain abnormality that underlies a tic disorder.

There are reasons why medical science has not yet found a single explanation for a tic disorder. People may develop tics for different reasons. Since tics are so common in children, we may all have a "gene for tics." However, the gene might have different expressions depending on the person. Recent studies have suggested that tics likely arise through the abnormal function or rearrangement of circuits deep within the brain. Learning a new complex task, such as playing basketball, requires changes within deep brain circuits that help the learner remember the task. Perhaps these brain circuits become poorly regulated by different genes, which then promote and enhance the repetition of unwanted movements and vocalizations. As discussed further in the book, the proper function of these deep brain circuits depends on many thousands of brain cell connections, each of which depends on many different types of brain chemicals called neurotransmitters. Breakthroughs in research might soon be expected as laboratory tools and genetic studies become more sophisticated. While tics fade away in most children without treatment, cognitive behavioral approaches, medications, or both can positively manipulate these deep brain circuits and supply relief from the tics.

What Causes the Tics?

For years physicians and scientists have searched for the cause of tic disorders. All kinds of tests and experiments have been performed, yet nothing abnormal has been found in the brains of affected people. There are a few hints that might shed light on the distinguishing characteristics or differences that might affect future clinical and scientific investigations: (1) tics are very common, so the difference is likely shared by many people; (2) imaging studies are normal, so the difference is very small; and (3) tics have a lot in common with habits, suggesting that the two might involve similar brain circuits. More hints can be found by closely examining the tics themselves.

Tics occur in response to a premonitory urge. The urge is a brief and odd sensation that is relieved by the tic. It is called "premonitory" because the urge occurs just before the tic. Young children do not generally notice the premonitory urge or the tic. Older children and adults who detect the premonitory urge have difficulty describing the sensation. So, what is this premonitory urge, and where does it come from? An answer may come from our knowledge of how habits are formed.

Habits are behaviors that are paired with cues. A cue is a signal, like a traffic light, that tells us what to do next. When a cue occurs, it can trigger a particular behavior. For example, a person walking into the kitchen may begin to feel hungry. In this case, the cue (walking into the kitchen) is paired with the habit (eating). However, the person may be unaware of either the cue or the habit. Recognizing the cue and the habit is essential to ending unwanted behavior.

Similar to habits, tics are also paired with cues. The cue is an internal feeling, referred to as a premonitory urge, which occurs just before the tic (fig. 1.1). About 70 percent of people with tics report feeling an urge just before the movement or sound.[1] The child with a tic disorder may begin to recognize the urge as they become older and

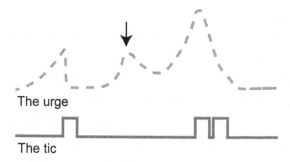

Figure 1.1 The urge and the tic. The illustration shows that the build in the urge (*dashed line*) is relieved by the tic (*solid line*). The second urge (*arrow*) is ignored. When the urge returns for the third time, it takes two tics to supply relief.

become more self-aware. The urge is difficult to describe; it is sometimes referred to as a pressure, a tightness, or an itch that is relieved by the tic. If the urge is noticed by younger children, they may call it a "pain" owing to a lack of another term to describe the sensation. One urge seems to require one tic. The urge subsides if it is ignored. However, the urge soon returns with greater power. A buildup in the number of unaddressed urges may result in a flurry of tics that occur one after another. In this way, the disorder takes on the counting characteristics of an obsessive-compulsive behavior. The repeated pattern of unwanted urges (obsessions) becomes more difficult to deal with and leads the person to perform repetitive behaviors (compulsions) called tics. The counting is subconscious, as a person with tics may not recognize it. As the child ages and becomes more aware of their condition, they may fight the urge as a way to suppress a tic in school. When the child relaxes upon returning home from school, the built-up urges trigger a flurry of tics that occur one after the other. A flurry of tics is sometimes called a tic storm. The astonished parent is left thinking that the child has been in such a state all day. When asked, however, their teacher may deny ever seeing or hearing a tic.

Are Tics a Habit?

A habit is a behavioral routine that has become nearly or completely involuntary. Certainly, a tic disorder fits neatly within the description of a habit. Like other habits, tics are primarily involuntary, can be suppressed, and occur in response to a premonitory urge. Like habits, tics can be controlled by cognitive behavioral therapies, including habit recognition and substitution or comprehensive behavioral therapy for tics. However, while tics are very similar to habits, they do not necessarily begin similarly. The "typical" habit is formed by someone who willingly and repetitively takes part in a specific behavior. The child never asked for the tic, and the movements began unconsciously. However, the overlap between tics and habits supplies some insight into what might cause the disorder and how it might be treated. Interestingly, while tics take on many aspects of a habit, persons with chronic motor and vocal tic disorder seem to have a lower risk of developing a substance use habit than the general population.[11]

What Causes the Urge and the Tic?

Since Gilles de la Tourette's research, many studies have been performed on persons with tics.[12] Despite the extraordinary efforts of many physicians and scientists, the cause of tic disorders remains unclear. As shown in box 1.1, there are at least four current theories. There is evidence that changes in genetic DNA might cause tics in certain families. Some physicians believe that tics are caused by an autoimmune disease, though most others are unsure. Tics might be caused by changes in brain structure or brain function that are too small to be seen on particular tests. Other clinicians believe that a tic disorder is a psychological condition since tics often occur alongside other psychological disorders.

Tic disorders are common diagnoses in children, and many others might have developed transient tics as children but do not remember them. Perhaps some people are more predisposed to develop tics than

BOX 1.1
Potential Causes of a Tic Disorder

Observations suggesting a genetic cause

- Inheritance patterns in some families
- Higher incidence of tics in brothers and sisters
- Overlap of symptoms with genetic causes of chorea
- No apparent changes in brain structure
- No identified antibodies

Observations suggesting an autoimmune cause

- Overlap in symptoms with chorea caused by rheumatic fever
- Observations suggesting that antibodies might alter brain chemical (neurotransmitter) receptors

Observations suggesting a developmental disorder that is caused by changes in brain structure or function (plasticity)

- Typical age of onset
- Imitation of tic-like movements by others
- Positive response to medications that are known to change neurotransmitters or their receptors
- Tics induced by drugs that enhance neurotransmitter availability; for example, cocaine may cause tic-like movements by increasing dopamine release
- Tics are reduced by drugs that block dopamine receptors

Observations suggesting a primary psychiatric disorder

- Association with other co-occurring psychological conditions
- Symptoms can overlap with a functional movement disorder
- No detectable abnormalities are seen on brain imaging or EEG studies

others. The same can be said of habits; some people are prone to bad habits, while others are not. Similarly, some of us are more anxious, obsessive, or compulsive. Some are more inattentive than others. These behaviors contribute to our personality and are part of the human equation. So which part of the brain might produce tics and help determine how we behave? Research suggests that the basal ganglia, structures deep within the brain, are responsible for learned movements, behaviors, habits, and addictions.

What Causes Habits?

While we know little about the brain mechanisms that might cause tics, we know much about what causes habits. The brain's outer surface, called the cortex, allows for conscious thoughts and planned activities.[13] A deeper part of the brain, called the basal ganglia, allows for learned movements and behaviors to occur automatically. The basal ganglia are needed so that we can think about other things as we walk, drive, or ride a bike. As we learn to do different things, the basal ganglia are programmed by a neurochemical called dopamine. Dopamine is released from nerve terminals into the basal ganglia when the subject is exposed to new situations.[13-15] Dopamine can then remodel brain areas specifically used to program motor movements.[13] When expanded to humans, these studies imply that dopamine, along with other brain chemicals, acts to program automatic motor functions that are needed for sports activities, writing, and the like.[16]

When first learning a skill, the actions are complicated and require the learner's full attention. With practice, the behavior or the series of movements and reactions is ingrained into the nervous system. Many adaptations in the brain are needed to learn a new skill. After a lot of practice, someone can successfully and automatically complete a very difficult task while focusing on other activities. For example, a person first learning to drive a car is fully engaged in the task. After a lesson or two, the activity becomes more automatic. With more practice, the person can soon engage in other simultaneous actions, such as eating or talking to a passenger. Of course, some people might be better learners than others. Some people will never be great skiers even if they take lessons and practice long and hard. Scientific evidence shows that the basal ganglia help to program these new learned skills.[17] The basal ganglia also take part in the generation of habits and diseases that affect dopamine release.[14,18] Indeed, the medications used to treat tics target the basal ganglia and its connections with other brain areas.[16] Small but essential changes in basal ganglia function may therefore account for differences in acquiring specific skills and developing certain behaviors, such as habits and tics.

Can Science Help Find the Cause of Tics?

It can be difficult to understand the workings of a child's mind. How do brain signals differ between a child with tics and one without? Scientists can answer these questions by studying certain behaviors. Models are then used to explore the origin of these behaviors. While there are no good models for tics, there are good models for habits. Models of dependence show that habits are characterized by tolerance and physiological symptoms upon withdrawal.[19] Tics share many similar features with habits, as they involve a premonitory urge and subsequent behavior, which helps to relieve the urge. Like tics, the urge associated with a habit can build up, resulting in the need to perform the task several times to make up for any missed tics. Arguably, tics move well beyond the typical behaviors accompanying routine habits and can cause a disruption of everyday activities and relationships.

How Do Brain Cells Communicate with Each Other?

This section will briefly explain how brain cells communicate with each other and how brain function can be modified by medication. The brain controls movements and behaviors using chemicals called neurotransmitters.[16] A neurotransmitter acts as a messenger so that one brain cell can communicate with another. When a brain cell becomes activated, it releases a neurotransmitter. The neurotransmitter flows across a small space called a synapse, where it binds to its receptor on the next cell (fig. 1.2). Like a railroad, the train (neurotransmitter) leaves the first station (brain cell #1) and travels down

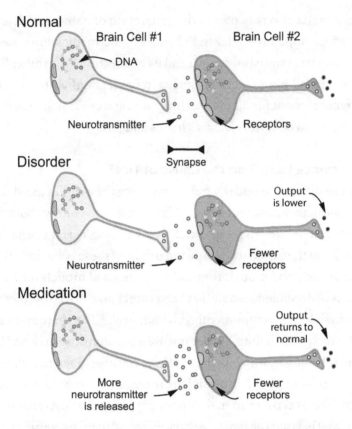

Figure 1.2 Medications can change brain circuits. *Top*: Brain cell #1 communicates with target brain cell #2 by releasing a neurotransmitter. The neurotransmitter binds to its receptor on the second cell. *Middle*: In some diseases, brain cell #2 may not make enough neurotransmitter receptors, in which case it does not work correctly when brain cell #1 makes the same amount of neurotransmitter. *Bottom*: Medication allows brain cell #1 to deliver more neurotransmitters, which compensates for the lower number of receptors on brain cell #2.

the track (synapse) to the platform (receptor) of the next station (brain cell #2). In this way information carried by the neurotransmitter can move across the brain.

There are many kinds of neurotransmitters in the brain. A neurotransmitter called glutamate activates cells. Another neurotransmitter called gamma-aminobutyric acid (GABA) inhibits cells. If a brain cell releases glutamate, the next cell is excited and information flows across the brain (the train conductor holds up a green arrow). If a brain cell releases GABA, the next cell is inhibited, and the signal stops (the conductor holds up a stop sign). Like a gas stove with a range of heat settings, brain function requires more sensitivity than on or off. Therefore, other neurotransmitters, such as dopamine and serotonin, act to make small adjustments in brain function.

Dopamine and serotonin are also called neuromodulators, as they supply relatively weak regulation of brain activity.[20] These brain chemicals participate in learning and can fine-tune movements and emotions. For example, dopamine may be released into the brain when a new situation is encountered.[13-15] If this situation occurs over and over, the repetitive release of dopamine promotes a long-lasting change in the brain that encourages learning and changes behavior.[21,22] If too much dopamine is released, the target cell may become overstimulated.[23] The number of dopamine receptors on the target cell will decrease to obtain a balance. A reduction in the number of receptors produces withdrawal symptoms when dopamine release falls to normal levels. Like a plant (the cell), too much water (dopamine) will cause the roots (receptors) to become shallow and weak. If the overwatering stops, then the plant is unable to thrive. Medications can help to regulate these neuromodulators, but changes in the receptors can be long-lasting.

It is becoming clear that changes in dopamine availability support habits.[14] Changes in dopamine, as well as other neuromodulators like serotonin, may underly neuropsychological disorders such as tics, anxiety, obsessive-compulsive disorder, and attention-deficit/hyperactivity disorder. These disorders can be treated, but they are difficult to cure. The medications used to treat these disorders change the brain circuits that produce these conditions, but they do not change the underlying cause. This may explain why an antipsychotic medication, such as haloperidol, that blocks dopamine receptors can help to reduce the number of tics.[24-26] Similarly, medications called selective serotonin reuptake inhibitors (or SSRIs) increase the amount of serotonin in the brain and are effective treatments for anxiety and obsessive-compulsive disorders.[27,28] Likewise, stimulant medications are thought to improve attention, as they increase brain dopamine levels.[29,30]

CHAPTER 2

Diagnosing
Tics and
Tourette's Disorder

The diagnosis of a tic disorder is made based on the person's symptoms. In this case, the symptoms are the movements and/or sounds that the person makes. No special blood or physiological tests, such as magnetic resonance imaging (MRI) or an electroencephalogram (EEG), can be used to diagnose a tic disorder.

A tic disorder is called a "neuropsychological condition," as the brain causes a change in behavior. Other specialists consider a tic disorder to be a "mental disorder," as it is a behavior that may cause distress or impairment in personal functioning.[1] Several diagnostic terms for tics have been developed and published in the *Diagnostic and Statistical Manual of Mental Disorders* (*DSM-5*; see box 2.1). The diagnoses in the latest *DSM-5* that relate to tics include provisional tic disorder, persistent (chronic) motor or vocal tic disorder, and Tourette's disorder. One more diagnostic category, called "other specified and unspecified tic disorders," is reserved for persons with tics who do not easily fit within the other categories. Other medical terms professionals use include Tourette's syndrome, transient tics, and chronic motor and vocal tic disorder. The diagnostic criteria that are outlined in the *DSM-5* are somewhat fluid and primarily based on the duration of symptoms and whether the symptoms include repetitive movements and/or vocalizations. For example, a person who has had motor and

BOX 2.1
Diagnostic Criteria for Tic Disorders

Provisional tic disorder

- One or more motor tics (e.g., blinking or shrugging the shoulders) or vocal tics (e.g., humming, clearing the throat, or yelling out a word or phrase)
- Tics have been present for no longer than 12 months in a row
- Tics started before the age of 18 years
- The person has symptoms that are not due to taking medicine or other drugs or to having a medical condition that can cause tics (e.g., Huntington's disease or post-viral encephalitis)
- The person has not been diagnosed with Tourette's disorder (Tourette's syndrome) or persistent motor or vocal tic disorder

Persistent (chronic) motor or vocal tic disorder

- One or more motor tics (e.g., blinking or shrugging the shoulders) or vocal tics (e.g., humming, clearing the throat, or yelling out a word or phrase) but *not* both
- Tics occur many times a day, nearly every day, or on and off throughout a period of more than a year
- Tics started before the age of 18 years
- The person has symptoms that are not due to taking medicine or other drugs or to having a medical condition that can cause tics (e.g., seizures, Huntington's disease, or post-viral encephalitis)
- The person has not been diagnosed with Tourette's disorder (Tourette's syndrome)

Tourette's disorder

- Two or more motor tics (e.g., blinking or shrugging the shoulders) *and* at least one vocal tic (e.g., humming, clearing the throat, or yelling out a word or phrase), although they might not always happen at the same time
- Have had tics for at least a year; the tics can occur many times a day (usually in bouts) nearly every day or off and on
- Tics started before the age of 18 years
- The person has symptoms that are not due to taking medicine or other drugs or to having another medical condition (e.g., seizures, Huntington's disease, or post-viral encephalitis)

Adapted from the Centers for Disease Control and Prevention. Diagnosing tic disorders. https://www.cdc.gov/ncbddd/tourette/diagnosis.html.

vocal tics for over a year can be diagnosed with Tourette's disorder. As discussed in the next section, it is unclear whether a diagnosis of Tourette's disorder really helps the patient.

Are Special Tests Needed to Diagnose Tics?

Once parents notice the movements or sounds of a child with tics, they often become concerned and seek medical attention. Occasionally, the pediatrician or family practice provider can rapidly make a diagnosis and supply counseling. As tics are often self-limited, the clinician usually delivers reassurance, and medical follow-up is arranged. However, tics such as repetitive blinking, coughing, or sniffing may initially pose a diagnostic challenge for the clinician. This can result in referrals to subspecialists, such as ophthalmology, pulmonary, or allergy medicine. Those with severe or atypical symptoms may be referred to see a neurologist. Atypical presentations or a concern that the symptoms might be seizures or even a brain tumor may lead to probing studies, including blood work, an EEG, or an MRI. The ability of the child to stop the movements, even for just a few seconds, indicates that the actions may be caused by a premonitory urge that is being suppressed for a few moments. The ability to transiently suppress the movements suggests that they are not caused by a severe disease that could be found by such testing. While testing is called for in some cases, such investigations might be limited, as the stress of medical testing will not likely help the child's symptoms.

It is important to know that EEGs and MRI can find issues that are unrelated to the tics. The EEG might show "slowing" or "spiking." The MRI might show unusual white spots, prominent blood vessels, or small cysts. These discoveries are often called "incidental findings," as they are often seen in the population and are unrelated to the tic symptoms. They can be a cause of concern to the parent and patient. The EEG and MRI are expected to be normal in someone with a tic disorder. If testing is performed, the parent should discuss the findings with the ordering clinician before jumping to any conclusions.

Incidental finding on an MRI scan

A 6-year-old girl developed blinking movements, and she seemed to be very anxious at times. Her doctor was concerned and ordered a brain scan. The MRI scan showed a normal brain, but there were a few scattered white spots. The child was then referred to a neurologist, who diagnosed the girl with a provisional motor tic disorder. He confirmed that the spots were "incidental" findings. He noted that the spots are often seen on MRI scans and are unrelated to the tics.

Why isn't there a medical test for a tic disorder? Brain imaging scans, such as MRI, have become highly advanced. However, even the best MRI scan cannot find neurochemicals and receptors in the brain. The standard 3-tesla-strength magnet in an MRI scanner resolves details of the brain down to about 1 millimeter.[2] While this seems incredible, a cubic millimeter of the brain contains about 50,000 brain cells, each establishing 6,000 contacts with neighboring brain cells.[3] Imaging studies, therefore, cannot visualize the tiny microscopic connections between cells.

Since many psychological disorders may be caused by changes in the connections between brain cells, other attempts have been made to measure neurotransmitters and their receptors.[4] An electron microscope can see neurotransmitter receptors in specially prepared brain slices. Of course, this technique is not practical for living people. These and other methods used to find the cause of tics have been inconsistent because medications and other factors can change brain connections and receptors. While prior investigations that specifically targeted the cause of tics have been disappointing and, at times, conflicting, the development of new scientific methods holds promise for future discoveries.

Does My Child Have Tourette's Disorder?

Tics are very common in children. According to one study, about 20 percent of children develop transient tics.[5] This may seem like a high percentage, but the number may be underestimated, and large-scale studies are needed.[6] Perhaps a much higher percentage of children develop transient tics, which rapidly disappear, never to be noticed by either child or parent. A much smaller number of children develop persistent chronic motor and/or vocal tics that can last for months or even years. Just 1 in 200 (0.5 percent) will develop chronic motor and vocal tics.[7] Therefore, about 0.5 percent of children meet the diagnostic criteria for Tourette's disorder, a mixture of motor and vocal tics that have been ongoing for more than a year.[5] It is important to realize that the diagnosis of Tourette's disorder does not consider the frequency and severity of the movements and vocalizations. People with a formal diagnosis of Tourette's disorder may be entirely dissimilar. For example, one person may have only occasional motor and vocal tics, while another may be much more affected. Furthermore, because simple vocalizations involve movements of the chest and throat, these sounds might arguably be referred to as motor tics rather than vocal tics.

The diagnosis of Tourette's disorder does not consider the presence of other psychological disorders that can occur in children with tics. These co-occurring conditions—anxiety, obsessive-compulsive disorder (OCD), and attention-deficit/hyperactivity disorder (ADHD)—can considerably affect a person's ability to learn and function in society. For instance, a person with tics can attend school, learn, and get a job. They can become an attorney or a professor. At the same time, someone with severe anxiety, OCD, or ADHD may be unable to leave the house or compete with other students in their class.

Therefore, the diagnosis of Tourette's disorder describes the type and duration of tic symptoms and does not imply that the child has suddenly developed a new and dangerous disease. In a sense, the diagnosis of Tourette's disorder can be stigmatizing, especially when the burden of tics is low. A diagnosis of Tourette's disorder does little to help the person with tics or their family. It does not alter treatment strategies or supply access to special services. Instead, the *DSM-5* criteria lump those with tics into broad descriptive categories that aid with clinical research and documentation. On the other hand, some persons who do meet the requirements for Tourette's disorder might be at greater risk of developing lifelong tics and other learning disorders.

A diagnosis of Tourette's disorder

A 14-year-old girl was referred to a neurologist for evaluation of her tic disorder. Her parents had noted blinking some years before. The pediatrician had told her parents that she had motor tics and not to worry, as the blinking would soon disappear. The blinking eventually stopped, but a few years later the parents noted occasional shoulder-shrugging movements, and about once a week they heard throat-clearing noises. The pediatrician diagnosed her with Tourette's disorder. The parents were upset and worried, as they had seen a television show about children with Tourette's who had persistent tics that were resistant to medication. The neurologist reassured the parents, noting that many people with a diagnosis of Tourette's disorder have mild tics that come and go.

Are Tics Dangerous, and Will They Disappear?

Tics generally develop between 4 and 6 years of age, but the age of onset varies widely.[8] Tics occur in boys more often than girls, at a ratio of four boys for every girl.[9] Initially, the tics are most often motor movements that involve the face, head, and shoulders. Occasionally, vocal tics will develop. On rare occasions, vocal tics might begin before the motor movements. Motor and vocal tics may occur together or in isolation. The tics come and go and change in type and intensity. For example, shoulder shrugging may be replaced by sniffing. Sniffing can then be replaced by blinking. Several motor and vocal tics can occur at different times, or they might occur simultaneously. Frequently the tics will stop unexpectedly. Sometimes the tics will stop entirely and come back weeks or months later for no clear reason.

The motor tic involves a brief, uncontrollable, spasm-like movement. These motor tics can produce muscle fatigue and pain due to muscle overuse when repetitive and frequent. This is a concern when the tics include abrupt head and neck movements. The vocal tics may attract more attention from bystanders. When occurring together, the verbal tics draw attention to the motor tics, and collectively they become more of a burden for the child.

Fortunately, most children have transient tics that disappear. The peak tic severity usually occurs between the ages of 10 and 12 years, with many children experiencing an improvement in tics in adolescence.[10,11] A longitudinal study that looked at persons with tics over a long period of time demonstrated that tic severity declined yearly during adolescence.[9] In this study, 18 percent of adolescents older than 16 years had no tics and 60 percent had minimal or mild tics six years after their initial examination. A much smaller number of children will develop a prolonged motor and/or vocal tic disorder that will persist into adulthood.[12–14] A very small number of children with tics will go on to develop more complex movements and vocalizations. Between 20 and 40 percent of those with chronic motor and vocal tics may develop complex motor and vocal tics, including copropraxia (inappropriate gestures) and coprolalia (repetitive offensive vocalizations).[15] While the research suggests a good outcome for most children with a tic disorder, it is difficult to predict which person with a tic disorder will go on to develop complicated and lifelong tics.

Do Tics Harm the Brain or Body?

There is no evidence that repeated tics are harmful to the brain. However, tics may cause embarrassment to the patient and their family or challenges with in- or out-of-school activities. On rare occasions, they may lead to orthopedic issues and muscle pain, caused by rapid and repeated head thrusting or head rotation movements. Over time, these tics can cause a repetitive use injury to the neck, similar to carpal tunnel, writer's cramp, or tennis elbow. Such prolonged and repeated head-moving tics may eventually require X-rays of the neck to ensure no secondary damage. This is an infrequent event, but medication to help reduce the tics is often needed under such circumstances.

Does Family History Matter?

Tics are very common in childhood, so finding another family member with tics, or a history of tics, is not surprising. Family members may have anxiety, obsessive-compulsive behaviors, or difficulties maintaining attention. While these conditions can occur in persons with a tic disorder, they are also very common behaviors in people. Interestingly, the brothers and sisters (siblings) of children with a tic disorder have a much higher frequency of developing the disorder. A recent study showed that a child has a 10 percent chance of developing Tourette's disorder if a sibling also has the disorder.[7] It remains unclear whether this higher rate, compared to 0.5 percent in the general population,[7] is due to genetics, imitation, or mimicking of the movements and/or sounds of their sibling, or other factors. Genetic studies have yet to find a single gene that causes tics in every affected person. Over the past 15 years, genetic studies have considered many different genes that might have produced the disorder in multiple individuals. There have been at least two studies that found a gene that caused the disorder in different families.[16] However, genetic variants known as "Tourette's risk genes" account for less than 2 percent of affected individuals.[17] Therefore, we still lack a genetic test that confirms the diagnosis or tells whether a family member is at risk for developing the disorder. While the family history is interesting and informative, it can only suggest that the tics and other co-occurring conditions have been passed down through the family.

My father has tics

A 15-year-old boy was seen in the neurology clinic for evaluation of his tics. He developed blinking and squinting movements when he was 6 years old. The tics never really bothered the boy, and the parents were not overly concerned. The boy told the doctor that his father also had tics. His father had a history of similar tics, but he claimed that the tics stopped some years ago. The boy's mother disagreed. She told the doctor that the father continued to have tics, but they did not happen all that often, and when they did, the father didn't seem to notice them.

Why Does My Child Not Seem to Recognize the Tics?

Simple tics, such as blinking, are often unrecognized by a person with a tic disorder. How can this be? Perhaps not recognizing a tic can be attributed to self-awareness. Self-awareness is the ability to accurately judge one's own performance and behavior and respond appropriately to different social situations. Self-awareness, along with other aspects of child development, grows over time. For example, between 4 and 5 years of age, children may start to pick out clothes they want to wear to school. Later, they may straighten up their room before friends come to play. They may begin to comb their hair and brush their teeth without prompting. When reaching 7 years of age, children with persistent tics may begin to notice the movements, and they may try to suppress the tics when they are in public. They do not want to be embarrassed by these movements and sounds when they are around friends. People are generally more self-aware of their actions in public. When not around others, people may become relaxed, become less self-aware, and do things that they would not ordinarily do when they are with friends. This may partially explain why tics occur more often when spending time alone, playing a video game, or watching television. The development of self-awareness may also play a role in explaining why some children stop having tics. They try hard to suppress the movements and develop behavioral approaches to block them; sometimes, these efforts pay off.

Self-taught comprehensive behavioral intervention for tics

The parents of a 5-year-old boy noticed that he seemed bothered by clothing that got close to his neck. He would pull his shirt collar down until he stretched the fabric and wrecked the shirt. Around the same time, the boy started to rub his chin against his chest. These activities would occur separately or together and were seen by his parents several times a week. He did not seem too bothered by any of it but did seem to enjoy stretching his shirts. After three years, the shirt pulling and head movements stopped and were replaced by another movement. The boy started using his left hand to gently scratch the underside of his chin. This movement was seen a few times a month and occurred in the evening before bedtime. He stopped stretching his shirts and began wearing ties when the social situation allowed. The neurologist concluded that the boy had a sensory aversion to the shirt collar and motor tics. The scratching movements were developed by the child as a way to block the tic. Sixteen years later the tics had not returned, but the boy continues to scratch his chin from time to time. The boy later recalled that he had eventually recognized the tics and developed the tic-blocking technique on his own.

How Can the Tics Simply Disappear?

Why do children sometimes have transient tics? Tics share characteristics with other habits that develop during a person's life. Some people may have a greater tendency to develop habits than others. Likewise, some people who develop bad habits can stop. For others, the habit can become an enduring and lifelong problem. Tics and habits share qualities. Behavioral approaches can be helpful if a person is aware of the behavior and is motivated to stop. Older children may develop techniques to help suppress the movements using methods quite similar, if not identical, to those used in comprehensive behavioral intervention for tics (see chap. 4). The older child has a better appreciation of the premonitory urge. Rather than making an urge-relieving tic, the child might make a deliberate alternative movement similar to the tic. This "fake" tic can quench the urge, and the tic may eventually disappear. Such self-taught behavioral therapy, called tic blocking, may help to reduce the frequency of tics and ultimately lead to a remission in symptoms. While it is impossible to accurately predict which child will go on to have persistent tics, the severity of tics during childhood and other psychological co-occurring disorders increases the likelihood of a prolonged or chronic condition.[13,14] Therefore, a comprehensive evaluation is needed. Treatment strategies should be carefully considered and tailored to the tic severity and the child's age.

CHAPTER 3

Associated
Conditions

Persons with tics are often well-behaved, are bright, and have good social skills. However, some people with a tic disorder can have one or more "co-occurring" psychological conditions or disorders. A co-occurring disorder means that a person with one disorder is more likely to have another. Tic disorder, anxiety disorder, obsessive-compulsive disorder (OCD), and/or attention-deficit/hyperactivity disorder (ADHD) often occur together, but the diagnoses are not necessarily made at the same time. These disorders are therefore referred to as co-occurring disorders. A co-occurring disorder is sometimes called a "comorbid" disorder. These disorders can change the person's ability to learn and function in school and other activities. There is a significant overlap between tics and these other three conditions (fig. 3.1). Heightened anxiety may increase the premonitory urge, causing the tics to worsen. Both OCD and ADHD can increase anxiety and the tics. Even if the symptoms of a co-occurring condition are mild, they can substantially impact the frequency and severity of the tics. Therefore, the identification and treatment of these conditions are necessary before the tics can be effectively treated.

Many if not all of us intermittently feel anxious. We may sometimes have obsessive-compulsive behaviors or challenges keeping attention. When the symptoms are severe and change one's ability to

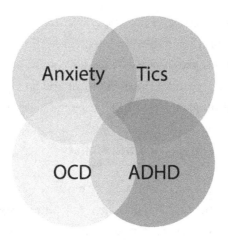

Figure 3.1 Many people with a tic disorder have another disorder as well, most commonly anxiety, obsessive-compulsive behavior, or inattention. Because these symptoms occur so frequently in persons with a tic disorder, they are called co-occurring conditions. Sometimes the symptoms of these co-occurring conditions are mild. When symptoms are severe, however, and detract from someone's life, that person might be diagnosed with anxiety disorder, obsessive-compulsive disorder (OCD), and/or attention-deficit/hyperactivity disorder (ADHD).

function properly, a clinician may diagnose the person with anxiety disorder, OCD, or ADHD. By the time a person is diagnosed with tics, they may or may not have already been diagnosed with one or more of these co-occurring conditions.

The symptoms of these co-occurring disorders will likely be present well before tics begin. Sometimes, upon reflection, the parents may have been suspicious that their child's behaviors were not quite right. For example, the child's parents might have wondered why their child was excessively fearful of leaving home or being left alone. Some parents might have been concerned about their child's poor attention span. Other parents might have wondered why their child had repetitive behaviors, such as touching objects repeatedly, or had become very upset when items or toys were out of a particular "correct" position.

It is important to realize that the symptoms of a co-occurring condition might be rather minor, in which case the person would not meet the diagnostic criteria for a "disorder." Nonetheless, the effective treatment of tics requires the evaluation and treatment of any co-occurring psychological condition if it seems to be affecting the tics.

Tics and anxiety

A 6-year-old girl was diagnosed with motor tics by her pediatrician. The tics didn't bother the girl, and they soon disappeared. However, at 10 years of age, the tics returned. She had developed shoulder-shrugging movements and throat-clearing sounds. The mother told the doctor that her daughter had occasional challenges coping with certain stressful situations, but this had never been a big problem. Her mother spoke to the schoolteacher and school counselor and discovered that her daughter was having a disagreement with another student. The tics stopped once the conflict was resolved.

What Are the Chances That a Person with Tics Has a Co-occurring Condition?

Research has shown that people with persistent motor and vocal tics are more likely to have a co-occurring condition. One study showed that only 15 percent of people with a tic disorder had isolated tics.[1] Therefore, one might assume that about 85 percent of people with chronic motor and vocal tics will display symptoms of a co-occurring condition. However, the chance of having a co-occurring condition seems quite variable across research studies in various populations. In one survey, between 38 and 60 percent of persons with Tourette's disorder also had ADHD.[2] Between 11 and 66 percent of those with Tourette's disorder also had OCD. The survey also showed that about

60 percent of those with Tourette's disorder had two or more of these co-occurring disorders. Nevertheless, while these disorders seem to occur together with some frequency, having one disorder does not necessarily mean that another condition will eventually develop. For example, people with tics may not have issues with anxiety. They may not show obsessive-compulsive behaviors or have challenges with keeping attention. Likewise, those persons with anxiety, with obsessive-compulsive behaviors, or who have challenges with keeping attention may not develop tics. So, while the data are mixed and sometimes confusing, screening for these co-occurring conditions in a comprehensive evaluation is necessary since finding and addressing a co-occurring psychological condition may help to reduce the tic burden.

Why Are Tics Associated with Other Psychological Disorders?

Sometimes persons with tics will also manifest symptoms of anxiety, OCD, and/or ADHD. While the cause of these disorders is currently uncertain, they all share similar brain circuits. The brain's outer layer, called the cortex, allows humans to think, plan, and move. Different areas of the cortex serve different purposes (fig. 3.2). For example, the brain's "motor cortex" helps to control movements. The "orbitofrontal cortex" processes sensations, rewards, and punishments. Another part of the cortex, called the "amygdala," manages emotions. Signals from the entire brain cortex are processed in the "basal ganglia." The basal ganglia lie beneath the cortex, where they help to support movements, learning, habits, behaviors, and emotions. Changes in how the basal ganglia process information from the cortex may cause a psychological disorder. Future research will help to show how changes in basal ganglia function might result in a tic disorder or a co-occurring psychological disorder. This crucial work is expected to explain how psychological disorders can develop and offer new and more effective treatment options.

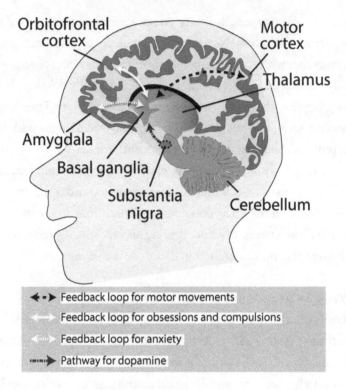

Figure 3.2 The basal ganglia serve as a memory bank for movements and behaviors. The illustration shows some important feedback loops that connect parts of the brain's outer surface, called the cortex, with the basal ganglia, a deep brain structure. A change in the loop from the motor cortex to the basal ganglia (*black dashed line*) may, theoretically, produce tics. Changes in the circuit to the orbitofrontal cortex (*white solid line*) may cause obsessive-compulsive behaviors. Changes in the circuit to the amygdala (*white dashed line*) may cause anxiety. Improper amounts of dopamine coming from dopamine-producing cells in the substantia nigra (*dashed oval*) may produce symptoms of attention-deficit/hyperactivity disorder. Also shown is a structure called the thalamus, which processes sensations. The cerebellum, which lies in the back part of the brain below the cerebrum, helps to coordinate movements and emotions.

Why Does Treating a Co-occurring Disorder Help to Reduce Tics?

The typical age of diagnosis for a co-occurring disorder is between 4 and 10 years.[1] Many children with a tic disorder experience the symptoms of anxiety. Anxiety is a feeling of fear, dread, and uneasiness. Anxiety is felt most when a person is in a stressful situation. In some ways, the premonitory urge feels like anxiety, and both are difficult for people to describe. The frequency and severity of the tics may increase in certain stressful circumstances. Therefore, the feeling of anxiety and the premonitory urge can crisscross so that heightened anxiety can feed the premonitory urge. In this way, anxiety associated with obsessive-compulsive behaviors or impaired attention can also increase the frequency of tics.

ADHD is often formally diagnosed between 6 and 8 years of age. However, the symptoms of ADHD are generally detected much earlier in childhood, and well before the onset of tics. Previously, it was thought that treating ADHD with stimulants such as methylphenidate (Ritalin) caused or "unmasked" the tics. However, recent evidence suggests just the opposite. The proper treatment of ADHD may also improve tic symptoms.[3] Stimulant medications may occasionally worsen tics in some patients with co-occurring ADHD. However, in a study done by the Tourette Syndrome Study Group, tic symptoms increased in 20 percent of participants who received methylphenidate, which was no more frequent than observed in participants who received a pretend medication, called a placebo (22 percent).[3] Therefore, the benefit of using a stimulant seems to outweigh the risk, provided that care is given to keeping the stimulant dose in the lower range.[2]

Tics and ADHD

A 9-year-old boy was referred to a neurologist for repeated nose-twitching movements. He had been an active boy in kindergarten and had difficulties focusing on schoolwork in first grade. His teacher became concerned. His pediatrician ordered testing and diagnosed the boy with ADHD. He was treated with a stimulant medication. His attention in the classroom and at home increased, and his school grades improved. About a year later the boy developed motor tics. The repetitive movements interfered with his ability to play baseball. His parents were concerned that the stimulant had caused the tics, but the tics worsened when the stimulant was stopped, and his school grades declined. It was felt that he was too young to take part in comprehensive behavioral intervention for tics. The neurologist suggested an alternative medication called guanfacine since, like the stimulant, it might help with both the tics and his ADHD symptoms. The tics improved, and he was able to maintain focus on his schoolwork.

Thus, it may come as little surprise that proper diagnosis and treatment of anxiety, obsessive-compulsive behaviors, and/or deficits in a person's ability to keep attention are needed before primary therapy for the tic disorder can begin. Again, it is important to realize that people with anxiety do not necessarily have an anxiety disorder and those with obsessive-compulsive behaviors may not meet criteria for OCD. Likewise, those who have trouble focusing on tasks do not necessarily have ADHD.

Children with a Tic Disorder Sometimes Have Problems with Speech, Sensations, Learning, and Sleep

Cognition is a term for the mental processes that take place in the brain. These mental activities include thinking, attention, language, learning, memory, and perception. Some children with Tourette's disorder may have challenges with speech, sensory processing, and/or learning. Other children with a tic disorder have challenges with sleep, which can affect learning.

A relatively low number of patients seen in the movement disorder clinic for tics also experience stuttering or other problems with speech. Stuttering, also called stammering, is a speech disorder that causes frequent problems with the smoothness and flow of speech. Another name for stuttering is a childhood-onset fluency disorder. People who stutter know what they want to say but have difficulty doing so smoothly, as they may repeat or prolong a word, a syllable, or a consonant or vowel sound. Stuttering is very common in children when they are learning how to speak. While most children outgrow this developmental stuttering, others do not. It can become a chronic condition affecting school performance, self-esteem, and interactions with others. Some important and famous people who have dealt with stuttering include US president Joe Biden, King George VI of the United Kingdom, and the author of *Alice in Wonderland*, Lewis Carroll. Developmental stuttering affects about 1 percent of the population. Stuttering may also be acquired. For example, "neurogenic stuttering" may occur after a substantial brain injury, and "psychogenic stuttering" can follow an emotional trauma.

Research reports show that stuttering can occur more often in people with a tic disorder. Still, the research outcome was sometimes based on small groups of people.[4,5] There may be reasons to assume that tics and stuttering are two co-occurring conditions, but this is probably not the case. Tic-like movements can occur in people who stutter, and those with vocal tics can make stuttering-like sounds. People with developmental stuttering produce more involuntary movements than others.[4] While some of these involuntary movements can be tics, other movements occur as a consequence of the stuttering. These secondary involuntary movements, such as forced eye closure, occur as the person tries to overcome the stutter. Challenges with verbal fluency certainly happen in people with tics; sometimes, their vocal tics resemble speech patterns seen in stuttering. Like tics, stuttering can often occur within families. Still, investigations have not been able to show a genetic link between the two disorders.[5] Treatment for stuttering includes speech therapy, cognitive behavioral therapy, or an electronic device to improve speech fluency.

Some children with a tic disorder have challenges dealing with certain textures or sensations. A person with sensory processing disorder (sometimes also referred to as sensory integration disorder) responds unfavorably to touch, taste, smells, sounds, or movements. Clothes may feel too tight, scratchy, or itchy. Sounds can be too loud, and light can be too bright. Soft touches feel hard, and certain food textures can make the person choke or gag. Most people dislike certain sensations, such as textures, sounds, and smells. People with a condition known as "misophonia" can get angry when they hear someone chewing. In excess, a dislike for certain sensations can affect the person's life, which can then be considered a disorder.

Sensory processing disorder can affect a considerable part of someone's day-to-day activities. Refusing to wear shoes, requiring a restricted diet, and other needs may affect the entire family. Significant challenges with sensory processing, such as touch aversion, are common in autism spectrum disorder. Sensory processing disorder is a controversial diagnosis and is not currently considered a stand-alone disorder. However, certain occupational therapists offer "desensitization" programs to help those with sensory processing issues. Desensitization is a treatment technique that normalizes the body's response to the sensation.

I can't wear my shoes

A 5-year-old boy with motor tic disorder was seen by his neurologist. The mother noted that the boy couldn't stand the feeling of socks and always refused to wear them. More recently, the boy stopped wearing shoes. The shoes made the boy feel "bad," and he cried when his parents tried to put them on. He wanted to go to school without shoes. The boy was sent to see a physical therapist, who tried different kinds of shoes. He liked the shoes with lights and agreed to wear those to school.

Like most people, those with a tic disorder are bothered by certain sensations. But some persons with a tic disorder will say that a sensation can provoke a tic. Tics may occur in response to specific environmental cues involving visual, auditory, and tactile stimuli. Tics can sometimes take the form of mirroring others' movements or vocalizations. Example cues include

- watching another person with tics;
- hearing certain words or sounds; and
- exposure to hot or cold temperatures.

A clinical study suggested that persons with chronic tics seem to have a slightly higher level of sensory intolerance (17 percent) than those without (6 percent), but the difference was insignificant.[6] Those with sensory intolerance may become distressed in response to external stimuli such as tags on clothes, elastic sock bands, and the sounds of others chewing. Like other disorders connected to tics, sensory intolerance might be more connected to OCD. Those with OCD are much more likely to have sensory intolerance (59 percent) than those without OCD (26 percent).[6] Overall, abnormal sensory processing can vary between persons but might occur more often in persons who have both a tic disorder and OCD. It is unclear how sensations might provoke a tic. As noted in chapter 1, the abnormal sensory function may theoretically account for the premonitory urge sensation that can occur just before the tic.

While most children with a tic disorder do well in school, others have challenges with learning. Many different neurological and psychological conditions can cause learning problems. Indeed, any medical condition that prevents students from listening to their teacher or doing their schoolwork will affect their learning ability. Conditions that affect learning may strongly affect a tic disorder. Difficulties at school can be caused by a short attention span or by a child who is easily distracted. A child may have obsessive-compulsive behaviors, where they must continue to repeat a task before moving on. Sometimes this involves reading the same word or the same line again and again. The anxious child may fear doing the wrong thing at the wrong time, so that nothing will get accomplished.

It is essential to consider other diagnostic possibilities in children with a learning disability. Important learning disorders that can be overlooked include dyslexia, dysgraphia, and dyscalculia. Dyslexia, dysgraphia, and dyscalculia describe specific problems with reading, writing, and arithmetic, respectively. It is essential to know that dyslexia, dysgraphia, and dyscalculia are not problems that affect a person's intelligence.

Dyslexia is a learning disorder that causes difficulty reading as a result of problems finding speech sounds and learning how they relate to letters and words. Signs of dyslexia can be difficult to recognize until the child learns how to read. When entering school, there can be word finding and pronunciation difficulties and challenges with reading, spelling, and processing what is read or heard. Early clues include the following:

- late in beginning to talk;
- learning new words slowly;
- reversing sounds in words or confusing words that look alike;
- difficulty learning rhymes; and
- problems naming or remembering colors or numbers.

Dysgraphia is a related learning disability that consists of illegible handwriting, inconsistent spacing, poor planning when composing a sentence or paragraph on paper, poor spelling, difficulty writing a composition, and challenges in thinking and writing simultaneously. Early clues include the following:

- difficulties holding and controlling a writing instrument;
- difficulties writing in a straight line;
- writing letters in reverse;
- difficulty recalling how letters are formed; and
- difficulty knowing when to use uppercase or lowercase letters.

Dyscalculia is a term used to describe a learning disorder that affects the child's ability to learn, understand, and perform mathematics and number-based operations. Children with dyscalculia have great difficulty learning and solving basic math equations like addition, subtraction, multiplication, and division. Children may also have challenges grasping concepts behind word problems and can struggle to understand graphs and charts. Early clues include the following:

- difficulties recognizing numbers and learning how to count;
- difficulties connecting numerical symbols with their corresponding word (e.g., 2 with *two*);
- using visual aids like fingers to help count; and
- difficulties recognizing patterns and placing items in certain orders.

The cause of dyslexia, dysgraphia, and dyscalculia is unknown. These conditions are thought to involve changes in the areas of the brain that process language. Their diagnoses are made by neuropsychological testing. Any brain changes related to dyslexia and dysgraphia are too small to be seen on a magnetic resonance imaging (MRI) scan or an electroencephalogram (EEG), and there are no special blood tests.

People with dyslexia have average intelligence and normal vision. However, convergence insufficiency, or the inability to move both eyes inward when reading, may mimic dyslexia. A medical provider can diagnose convergence insufficiency, but sometimes a complete examination by an ophthalmologist is needed. The degree of dyslexia, dysgraphia, and dyscalculia can vary widely between people. Those with more minor symptoms can sometimes remain undiagnosed. However, it is essential to assess for dyslexia and dysgraphia when people have difficulty reading, writing, and using numbers. Early assessment and intervention can be helpful.

Persons with tics can present with similar symptoms. Tics that involve the eye can make reading difficult. This is especially true when the tics involve blinking or eye-rolling. A psychoeducational evaluation or a neuropsychological assessment should be considered if a child is behind in their school class or has other identified problems learning or performing. A psychoeducational evaluation is often provided by the child's school upon request. Alternatively, a neuropsychological assessment can be obtained privately or through a large academic center. A neuropsychological assessment is similar to but more comprehensive than a psychoeducational evaluation.

People with a tic disorder may have problems falling or staying asleep. Studies that have examined the effect of sleep deprivation have found deficits in cognitive processing.[7] Therefore, it is important to determine why a child is having challenges with sleep and to address these issues. So why would a person with tics have sleep difficulties? Tics increase when the person is relaxing in the evening and perhaps engaged in an activity that requires little thinking, such as watching television or playing a video game. An increase in tics may also occur when the person is preparing for sleep and can affect the ability to fall asleep. Fortunately, tics are generally absent during sleep, but tics might resume if they wake during the night.

Other factors besides tics may also contribute to poor sleep. Ruminating about earlier daytime experiences or the feeling of anxiety associated with the next day's activities will keep many people awake. This will make it difficult to return to sleep if aroused during the night. Persons with obsessive-compulsive behaviors may need to wait until the "correct" time before allowing themselves to sleep. There are undoubtedly other factors that could cause poor sleep. Sometimes obtaining a complete history will supply important clues that can help find the problem. Other times, the person with tics will need to see a sleep specialist. A sleep study may determine the underlying cause. A sleep study can show obstructive sleep apnea, restless legs syndrome, and other disorders that are generally unrelated to tics.

Falling asleep in class

The teacher of a 10-year-old girl with tics told her mother that she had been falling asleep in class. The mother was concerned, as the girl was going to bed on time. The mother discovered that her daughter had gone to bed but not to sleep. She was up late into the night, messaging her friends and using social media. The girl told her mother she was nervous at bedtime and that her tics increased. Having difficulty falling asleep, she spent time on her tablet. The mother began reading to her daughter at bedtime, her electronic tablet was left in the kitchen, and the problem disappeared.

Accurately diagnosing the cause of poor sleep will help name interventions that can help. Going to bed at a particular time is a good idea. It will certainly help those with anxiety. The symptoms of anxiety increase when a typical routine is interrupted. The bed should generally only be used for sleeping. Reading or other relaxation exercises may have a calming effect and reduce the number of tics. Watching TV, texting, and social media should certainly be avoided. A simple alarm clock should be used rather than a smartphone, which should be kept in another part of the house. Generally, small but meaningful changes in behavior can help to reduce issues with sleep. If the problem is resistant to such efforts, the clinician may discuss medication. If tics awake the child, the clinician may suggest supplying a small dose of clonidine or guanfacine just before bedtime (see chap. 4). The child's clinician may also suggest diphenhydramine (Benadryl) or melatonin. Consultation with the clinician will help parents find the best strategies to try.

Other Psychological Conditions That Might Be Seen with Tics and a Co-occurring Condition

Anxiety, obsessive-compulsive behaviors, and attention-deficit/hyperactivity are considered co-occurring conditions, as a person with a tic disorder has a good chance of having one or more of these other issues. Several other conditions might occur in persons with tics, but the chances of having one of them are not very high. A few people with a tic disorder might also have an impulse control disorder or a disruptive behavior disorder such as conduct disorder or oppositional defiant disorder.[1,2] Some persons with tics may have depression or another mood disorder. Others may have autistic spectrum disorder, self-injurious behavior, or a personality disorder. As discussed below, these disorders may be more associated with anxiety, OCD, or ADHD than with tics.

An impulse control disorder refers to a condition where individuals may have difficulty properly controlling their impulses and behaviors or actions and reactions to stimuli.[8] Some examples of this disorder include breaking rules, stealing, disobedience, destroying property, angry outbursts, arguing, and fighting. This disorder includes five types of conditions: kleptomania, pyromania, intermittent explosive disorder, oppositional defiant disorder, and conduct disorder. Kleptomania and pyromania refer to conditions where the person feels an overpowering and irresistible urge to steal things and start fires, respectively. People with these conditions know that these things are wrong, and they may (or may not) feel remorseful after the fact, but they act to obtain a release from the urge. People with an intermittent explosive disorder have frequent episodes of impulsive anger toward people or animals that is out of proportion to the event that triggered it.

Impulse control disorders occur in 1–4 percent of the general US population. Their diagnosis requires an evaluation by a psychologist or a psychiatrist. Impulse control disorder is different from OCD. Impulsive behaviors are spontaneous actions. The person does think about the potential consequences of those actions. Compulsive behaviors are usually performed repeatedly to reduce emotional or physical discomfort and feel better.[9] There are no medications approved by the Food and Drug Administration for treating an impulse control disorder. An individualized treatment utilizing cognitive behavioral therapy and other methods is required.[8] An impulse control disorder seems to be more common in those with Tourette's disorder. This may be due to the presence of a co-occurring condition, as impulsivity generally increases with the presence of anxiety and ADHD.[10,11] The details, though, are unclear, as there are not many controlled studies in the area of impulse control and Tourette's disorder.[12] It is important to know that children can be impulsive and defiant at times. An impulse control disorder, in contrast, involves ongoing patterns of more severe behaviors.

Persons with disruptive behavior disorder show ongoing patterns of uncooperative and defiant behavior. It is usual for children to "act out" on occasion. Acts of defiance toward family members and parents are not uncommon. If dysfunctional behaviors become repetitive and last for more than six months, the child's parents should seek professional help. Disruptive behavior disorders include conduct disorder and oppositional defiant disorder. The two have similarities but significant differences. Both are related to ADHD, so they can occasionally be seen in children with tics.

Swearing in class

A 13-year-old boy with Tourette's disorder started screaming profanities in class. His teacher contacted the parent to complain. He had a history of making intermittent throat-clearing noises but had never used swear words. The boy blamed the tics. The school psychologist discovered that the boy's classmates had suggested that he yell to create a disturbance. The vocalizations soon stopped.

A conduct disorder can be diagnosed when someone displays inappropriate behaviors, aggression, or anger. A conduct disorder is a group of behavioral and emotional problems characterized by a disregard for others. Those with a conduct disorder have a difficult time following rules and behaving in a socially acceptable way. They may enjoy causing harm, lying, or manipulating others. They may commit physical or sexual violence and may enjoy hurting animals. They may actively defy or refuse to cooperate, and they can blame others for their own mistakes or misbehaviors. Notably, a person with tics and conduct disorder may purposely use their tics as an excuse to annoy others. When this happens, it can be difficult for the parent, teacher, and clinician to decide exactly why the person with tics is making loud noises or using profanities. Vocalizations that occur only in certain situations may show that the problem is related to a conduct disorder rather than a tic. Treatment of a conduct disorder includes family therapy, behavioral modification, and medications, often in combination. Fortunately, about 70 percent of those who display symptoms of conduct disorder will grow out of it by adolescence. Clinical investigations have shown that conduct disorder can occur in persons with tics. One recent study showed that conduct disorder occurs in about 15 percent of those with Tourette's disorder.[13] These findings suggest that a tic disorder and a conduct disorder are not co-occurring conditions. In other words, conduct disorder is probably not connected to a tic disorder. However, conduct disorder is related to ADHD, and it can be seen in persons with a family history of aggressive and violent behaviors.

Persons with oppositional defiant disorder are easily agitated and often lose their temper. They may express anger and resentment and tend to argue with anyone in authority. They purposefully disobey rules and partake in disruptive behavior. They tend to lay blame on others and can be spiteful or seek vengeance. These behaviors can vary between people; they can be mild or extreme. Oppositional defiant disorder is related to conduct disorder, but they have different qualities. Oppositional defiant disorder involves problems keeping control, while conduct disorder involves issues with being controlled and the need to exert control over others.

It is important to realize that persons with tics may have a higher rate of temper tantrums. People can occasionally get upset and "lose their temper" if they feel that a situation is out of control. This can often occur if a person with a tic disorder has anxiety, obsessive-compulsive behaviors, or ADHD. Those with OCD can become visibly upset if a particular ritual is interrupted. The feeling of anxiety can become overwhelming, and the person can lose physical and emotional control. Temper tantrums are sometimes profound enough that the term "rage attack" can be appropriate. Learning relaxation techniques and coping mechanisms that can be used at a moment's notice may help reduce periodic flairs in anxiety and the number of tantrums or rage attacks.

Depression and bipolar disorder are called mood disorders.[14] A mood disorder is a mental health condition that affects someone's emotional well-being and interferes with their ability to function properly. Their emotional state is distorted or inconsistent with the current circumstances of their life.

Depression is a common and serious medical illness that negatively affects how someone feels, the way they think, and how they act.[15] Persons with depression can have prolonged and persistent periods of extreme sadness. Depression is a common mood disorder and occurs in about 10 percent of adults in the United States.[16] Depression is also common in persons with chronic motor and vocal tics. Clinical studies have shown that depression occurs in about 13 percent of those with Tourette's disorder, and milder depressive symptoms may occur in up to 75 percent.[17] Depression in people with chronic tics has been shown to result in a lower quality of life, potentially leading to hospitalization and suicide.

People with bipolar disorder can also be depressed, but their mood cycles between depression and what is called mania.[18] A person with mania displays an over-the-top level of activity or energy, mood, or behavior. The elevation of mood is excessive and is noticed by others. They may feel invincible, stay awake for long periods of time without fatigue, and have racing thoughts or ideas. Speech can be rapid, and the person can express strange beliefs or perceptions. On rare occasions, individuals with tics may also have bipolar disorder, but it is unclear whether they are co-occurring conditions.

The underlying cause of depression and bipolar disorder is unclear. However, screening for a mood disorder during a clinic visit is recommended, as diagnosing these individuals and supplying proper psychological treatment can improve their condition.

Children with autism spectrum disorder can also develop a tic disorder. According to the Centers for Disease Control and Prevention, autism spectrum disorder is a developmental disability caused by brain differences.[19] These differences may be caused by a metabolic or genetic disorder, but most causes remain unclear. People with autism spectrum disorder may behave, communicate, interact, and learn in ways different from most others. The severity of the disorder varies widely among those with the diagnosis. Some with autism may be impaired and need help, while others require little or no support. The symptoms of autism spectrum disorder include problems with communication and social interaction, restrictive and excessive interests, specific sensory characteristics (hypo- or hypersensitivity), and repetitive behaviors. Learning and attention may be reduced. There are often impairments in eye contact with people they are communicating with. Some people with autism spectrum disorder dislike touching and are very sensitive to different textures and sensations. People have differences in how they communicate and interact with others. These differences are part of our personality. When these personality traits become excessive and affect day-to-day function, a psychological diagnosis of autism spectrum disorder might be made.

Autism spectrum disorder is another neuropsychological condition that has been reported to occur in persons with a tic disorder. Like those with a tic disorder, people with autism can have symptoms of anxiety, depression, ADHD, and obsessive-compulsive behaviors. Like the symptoms of autism spectrum disorder, these behaviors can be mild or can be severe and affect day-to-day functioning.

The indications of autism spectrum disorder can often be detected in early childhood, and a diagnosis by an experienced professional is possible by 2 years of age. If the symptoms are mild, the diagnosis might be delayed by many years. The diagnosis of autism spectrum disorder is made by neuropsychological testing. No extraordinary brain or blood tests can verify the diagnosis of autism spectrum disorder. Although the specific cause is unknown, risk factors for developing autism include a sibling with autism spectrum disorder, being born to older parents, and having certain genetic conditions.

There are overlapping features between autism spectrum disorder and a tic disorder. They share common co-occurring conditions, like anxiety and ADHD. However, there are differences. The diagnosis of autism spectrum disorder can be made by 2 years of age. The onset of tics occurs much later, around 4–6 years of age. Most abnormal movements in autism spectrum disorder are complex motor stereotypies, such as spinning and hand flapping. As discussed further on, stereotypies are repetitive movements that stay similar over time. Tics tend to wax, wane, and change over time.

Motor and vocal tics can undoubtedly occur in people with an autism spectrum disorder. Clinical studies have shown that people with autism spectrum disorder are more likely to develop tics than the general population.[20] A clinical analysis performed in 2017 showed that while some people with chronic tics may also have autism spectrum disorder, the cause of the two conditions may be quite different.[21] The investigators used the self-reported Social Responsiveness Scale, which evaluates social awareness, cognition, communication, motivation, restrictive interests, and repetitive behavior. Based on this particular test, about 23 percent of children and 9 percent of adults with chronic tics met the criteria for autism spectrum disorder. These numbers are much higher than in the general population, where only 0.3–2.9 percent of people without tics are diagnosed with an autism spectrum disorder. This seems to mean that people with chronic tics are more likely than others to have autism. However, the investigators concluded that the increased frequency of autism in people with chronic tics might reflect similar symptoms. Repetitive behaviors, deficits in attention, and obsessive and compulsive behaviors are common to both. Therefore, autism spectrum disorder and tic disorder may occur together but are likely two distinct disorders that share overlapping features. It is essential to know that someone who has autism spectrum disorder may have a higher likelihood of developing tics. On the other hand, someone who has tic disorder will not likely develop autism spectrum disorder later in life.

Some children with tics can also demonstrate self-injurious behaviors. These behaviors include cutting, head hitting, head banging, and self-biting. These behaviors can result in minor injuries such as bruises or scratches. Children with self-injurious behaviors rarely cause more severe injuries to themselves, such as blindness or broken bones. Similar to tics, self-injurious behaviors seem to be involuntary. However, there are reasons why someone would engage in self-injury. The behavior may result in increased attention or access to something they want, but it is important for the parent to know that the child may not realize this. Self-injurious behaviors are distinct from self-stimulatory behaviors and motor stereotypies that supply comfort for the person engaged in the activity. Self-injurious behaviors are not directly related to a tic disorder. However, they are typically associated with a learning disability or another neuropsychological condition, such as OCD and depression.[22] Self-injurious behaviors can be addressed by cognitive behavioral therapy and other treatments that focus on any other co-occurring psychological disorders.

People with a personality disorder can also develop a tic disorder. The *Diagnostic and Statistical Manual of Mental Disorders* lists 10 types of personality disorders: paranoid, schizoid, schizotypal, antisocial, borderline, histrionic, narcissistic, avoidant, dependent, and obsessive-compulsive.[23] These disorders include persistent and long-lasting patterns of unusual ways to feel, think, and behave. They do not allow the person to adjust adequately or appropriately to certain situations or to their surroundings. Persons with a personality disorder exhibit poor coping skills, have distorted perceptions of reality, and demonstrate inadequate behaviors.[24] Personality disorders lead to significant distress and dysfunction.[24,25] Personality disorders occur in about 6 percent of adults.[23] While children can show some symptoms of a personality disorder, usually a diagnosis can only be made in adults aged 18 and older.[26]

Several studies in adults have shown that those with Tourette's disorder have a higher frequency of personality disorders.[27] Similar to the other disorders listed in this chapter, the increased risk of having a personality disorder is largely due to the presence of a co-occurring condition, such as anxiety disorder,[28] OCD,[29] and ADHD.[30]

Anxiety is a common feature of several personality disorders. Avoidant personality disorder has much overlap with an anxiety disorder. As said before, anxiety is a feeling of fear, dread, and uneasiness.[31] Avoidant personality disorder is characterized by an excessive pattern of feelings of extreme social inhibition, feelings of inadequacy, and high sensitivity to negative criticism and rejection.[32] Both anxiety disorder and avoidant personality disorder can result in low self-esteem and self-isolation. Those with OCD are at risk of having an obsessive-compulsive personality disorder.[33] Obsessive-compulsive personality disorder is not the same as obsessive-compulsive disease, but the two may occur together. Obsessive-compulsive personality disorder is characterized by an excessive preoccupation with detail and orderliness, excessive perfection, and the need for control over one's environment.[33] OCD is characterized by repeated, persistent, and unwanted thoughts (obsessions) with or without compensatory actions (compulsions) that are unpleasant and cause distress or anxiety.[34] People with ADHD are at risk for having borderline personality disorder.[30] Those with borderline personality disorder have challenges with emotional regulation, interpersonal relationships, and self-image. Both those with ADHD and those with borderline personality disorder have difficulty with impulse control, as discussed above.

Most people show personality traits that would seem to fit into a personality disorder. However, those who are diagnosed with a personality disorder have severe symptoms that affect their ability to function in an ordinary way. They tend to always act and react the same way, and it is very difficult for them to adequately adjust their behaviors to different situations. A personality disorder is challenging to diagnose, and it is very difficult to treat.

Neurological Disorders That May Look Like Tics

Tics are common in children, and the patient's primary medical provider often diagnoses them. However, some tics are quite different, and the diagnosis can be challenging. Some tics may seem to come out of nowhere; in contrast, other tics develop in response to a repetitive movement or sound caused by a different problem. For example, a child may develop an environmental allergy or viral illness that produces a stuffy nose. The child begins sniffing, and this turns into a habit tic. The pediatrician may then send the child to see an allergist. Likewise, persistent cough or blinking might result in consultation with a pulmonologist or an ophthalmologist. Such referrals may be necessary to exclude disorders that require special treatment.

Tourette's disorder mimics another disease

An 8-year-old boy presented to his pediatrician with complaints of a persistent cough that had lasted over three months. His examination was normal, and no coughing occurred in the office. However, the cough persisted at home and at school, and he was referred to a lung specialist (pulmonologist). A chest X-ray, an MRI scan of the chest, and pulmonary function studies were performed. The tests were all normal. He did not seem to have asthma. He was sent to see an allergist. No reason for the cough could be found. Two months later, the mother noted repetitive blinking. The blinking was soon replaced by repeated shrugging of the shoulders.

At 10 years of age, he was seen by a neurologist, who diagnosed Tourette's disorder. No further tests were performed, and no medication was given. The coughing and blinking stopped the following year.

A child might occasionally present with abnormal movements that suggest tics, but the parent and clinician might be concerned about missing the correct diagnosis. If tics seem unlikely and if the movements are complex, other possibilities should be considered. There are many childhood-onset movement disorders.[35] Disorders such as complex motor stereotypies can be similar to tics, while other conditions, such as seizures, are generally very different. This section will discuss the more frequent movement disorders in children and explain why they differ from tics.

Various nonthreatening movement disorders can be seen in infancy and early childhood (box 3.1).[36] They are termed benign and developmental movement disorders of childhood owing to their favorable outcome and lack of other abnormal neurological findings on examination. These movements generally resolve spontaneously and entirely as the child ages.[36] However, the parent may become quite concerned, and the clinician might worry that the movements could be seizures. While some part of the movement might mimic a tic, they appear in children who are too young to develop a tic disorder.

Abrupt jerking of an arm or leg is common in a sleeping infant and is called benign sleep myoclonus. Sometimes the jerking movements occur when the baby is awake or feeding. The movements start in infancy, and the average age of resolution is about 1 year. Other odd movements can occur in infants. These include sudden or rhythmic movements of the arms or legs, periodic upward movements of both eyes, posturing of a limb or the head to one side, strange eye movements, and abrupt shuddering spells. On rare occasions, a par-

BOX 3.1

Unusual Movements in Childhood

Movement	Age of onset	Age when they often disappear
Benign paroxysmal torticollis	1 week to 30 months	<4 years
Benign sleep myoclonus	<2 weeks	3 months to 3 years
Complex motor stereotypies	<3 years	Up to adulthood
Gratification behavior	2 months to 6 years	Up to adulthood
Mirror movements	3–4 years	<7 years
Paroxysmal tonic upgaze	1 week to 5 months	<4 years
Sandifer syndrome	3 weeks to 14 years	No resolution if left untreated
Shuddering attacks	<1 year	<4 years
Sleep-related rhythmic movements	<3 months	Up to adulthood
Spasmus nutans	4–18 months	1–2 years after onset
Tic disorder	4–8 years	Up to adulthood
Transient dystonia of infancy	5–10 months	3 months to 5 years

Adapted from Bonnet C, Roubertie A, Doummar D, Bahi-Buisson N, Cochen de Cock V, Roze E. Developmental and benign movement disorders in childhood. *Mov Disord.* 2010;25:1317–1334.

ent might notice that their child has symmetrical movements of the hands. When one hand moves, the other will automatically do the same. The movements of concern generally stay the same, they can frequently be suppressed by manipulating the affected arm or leg, and they often disappear as fast as they started. Taking a short video recording of the movement while gently moving the affected limb can help the clinician find the diagnosis.

Funky baby movements

A 3-day-old infant was taken to the pediatrician for abrupt movements of the limbs. The movement was seen sometimes in an arm and sometimes in a leg. The movement would often occur when the baby was feeding and falling asleep. The doctor sent the baby to the local emergency room. The baby was admitted to the hospital for an EEG to help exclude seizures. The EEG was normal. A diagnosis of benign sleep myoclonus reassured the parents. The movements stopped a few months later.

A complex motor stereotypy is a frequent benign movement that begins in early childhood, and they are often confused with motor tics. Movements are stereotyped when they are involuntary, repetitive, rhythmic, suppressible with distraction, and seemingly purposeful in character but unusual in form and when they possess a predictable pattern, amplitude, and location.[37]

Stereotypies are often mislabeled as motor tics, but there are key differences. Like tics and habits, stereotypic movements are often subconscious, and there can be a cue and an urge. A cue, such as a sound, a reward, or a surprise, might provoke the stereotypic action. Older children with stereotypies might describe a premonitory urge, a feeling that the movement needs to happen. As the name suggests, the stereotypic movements generally stay the same over time. On the other hand, tics are dynamic: they shift from one action to another over days, weeks, or months. Another difference between tics and stereotypies is that stereotypies often first develop in very young children. Unlike tics, which usually begin between 4 and 6 years of age, motor stereotypies typically start within the first three years of life. In a group of normal children with complex motor stereotypies, about 80 percent of these started before 24 months, 12 percent between 24 and 35 months, and 8 percent at 36 months or older.[38]

Stereotypies

A 4-year-old girl had been making odd movements with her arms whenever she was excited. She would bring her hands up toward her mouth and bare her teeth. Her hands would tremble slightly. The movements would last just a second or two and seemed to be interruptible with distraction. While highly predictable and self-similar, they could occur dozens of times each day. Her development had been typical, and her neurological examination was reassuring. The girl was diagnosed with complex motor stereotypies. Later, mother and child spent time together in front of a large mirror. The mother showed the girl what she was doing that had brought the two of them to the doctor. Using only positive reinforcement, the mother intermittently encouraged her to do other things with her hands when she was excited.

Stereotypic movements are common, occur in various forms, and exist in different populations, ranging from typically developing children to those with autism.[37] Infants and young children tend to exhibit more complicated movements such as finger wiggling, hand flapping or rotation, arm flapping, head nodding, and body rocking. These are often called complex motor stereotypies. Stereotypies in older children and adults are often simpler and might include nail biting, tapping their feet, pencil spinning, hair twirling, and the like. About 20 percent of children show common and simple types of motor stereotypies. Complex motor stereotypies are estimated to occur in about 4 percent of the population.[38]

Stereotypic movements last from seconds to minutes, appear multiple times a day, and are associated with periods of excitement, stress, fatigue, or boredom. Each child has a certain repertoire, or collection of movements, which can very slowly evolve with time. Stereotypic movements may be combined with other behaviors, such as mouth opening, neck stretching, vocalizations, or sniffing. They can be readily suppressed by stimulation or distraction. Occasionally, children report that they enjoy performing the movement, although most children seem not to notice.

Similar to tics, stereotypies can be upsetting to parents. Parents may be concerned that the stereotypy will be disruptive, interfere with their child's ability to make friends, or result in other children's teasing or bullying. The movements, however, are usually of little concern to the child. Similar to tics, the frequency of ADHD, learning disabilities, or obsessive-compulsive behaviors is higher in typically developing children with complex motor stereotypies.[39] Secondary stereotypies most often occur in those with autism spectrum disorder.[39]

The diagnosis of a complex motor stereotypy is based on history and visual inspection. Tests such as brain MRI and EEG are unhelpful. Evidence-based therapy for the suppression of motor stereotypies is generally lacking, and the response of stereotypic movements to medications is largely inconsistent.[37] Behavioral interventions in the autistic population have been used with varying success. In typically developing children, the combination of habit reversal and differential reinforcement of other behaviors may be beneficial in reducing the frequency of motor stereotypies. Behavioral substitution and positive reinforcement are perhaps the best ways of producing a long-lasting reduction in stereotypies.[38] Cognitive behavioral techniques might be tried if the stereotypies worsen with time and age. This treatment works best with older children who can better appreciate the therapy and understand what the therapist asks them to do.

Functional Movement Disorders

Older children and adolescents who seem to have a tic disorder may instead have what is called a "functional" movement disorder. A functional movement disorder occurs when someone displays unusual and involuntary movements or body positions with no identifiable cause.[40] Functional movement disorders can manifest in many ways. Sometimes the movements can mimic severe neurological diseases such as dystonia or seizures. Rippling stomach muscles, intermittent ankle stiffness, and arm and leg posturing may come and go or persist for years. Walking can look bizarre and seem uncoordinated, but balance is maintained, and falls are rare. Convulsions with or without loss of consciousness can occur. Unlike epileptic seizures followed by confusion and tiredness, the patient may rapidly recover and return to baseline. Also contrary to epileptic seizures, biting of the lip or the side of the tongue and the release of urine or stool during the convulsion are often absent.

A functional movement disorder can also resemble a motor and vocal tic disorder. The onset of movements and vocalizations can be abrupt, relentless, and severe. It generally occurs in adolescents who seem too old to develop tics and have no history of prior tics. Swearing (coprolalia), inappropriate gestures (copropraxia), throwing objects, and self-abusive behaviors are common.

During the COVID-19 pandemic, there was a surge in adolescents, often girls, who presented to their clinician, or even to the emergency department, with an abrupt onset of motor and vocal tics. The increased frequency of functional movement disorders during the COVID-19 pandemic suggests that stress might contribute to the condition. There is mounting evidence that some of these persons were using social media.[41,42] Clinicians noted that their patients' movements are similar, if not identical, to videos posted on these social media platforms.[43] This suggests that the affected person may have been subconsciously imitating the movements of popular influencers.[41,42] Other clinical studies have indicated that many girls posting videos of their "tics" do not likely have tics.[43] This suggested that some of the girls posting their tic-like movements online pretend to have tics to raise awareness of the disorder or to get a following.

A functional movement disorder can be challenging for the clinician to diagnose initially. However, repeated clinical assessments can eventually help to secure the diagnosis. Separating a functional movement disorder from a severe case of tics can also be a challenge, as they share similar symptoms.[44] For example, the premonitory urge may be absent in persons with either tics or a functional movement disorder, and the sudden onset of tics that occurs in those with a functional movement disorder has been reported in adults with Tourette's disorder. Furthermore, someone with tics or a functional movement disorder may not have a family history of tics. Finally, self-injurious behaviors, the inability to suppress the tics, suggestibility with increased movements when discussing the tics, and a lack of response to well-established tic-suppressing medication may occur in people with either disorder. Similar to persons with tics, those with a functional movement disorder have normal EEG and brain imaging studies.

A functional movement disorder resembles a tic disorder

A 14-year-old previously healthy girl awoke one morning with a storm of unrelenting motor and vocal tics. She experienced repeated blinking, eye-darting, and mouth-opening movements. Sometimes an arm would fly up in the air, occasionally striking another person. She would hum, yell, and occasionally curse. Every few minutes she would extend her arm and her middle finger. This went on for two months, and eventually her mother decided to take her out of school. When asked, the girl noted that she watched videos on social media every day. She agreed that the movements and sounds seemed very similar to someone that she actively followed on a social media platform. It was agreed on that she would stop watching that person's videos. She was referred to a psychologist for further evaluation and was offered comprehensive behavioral intervention for tics. Six weeks later, the movements had stopped, and she was back in school.

Coming to a rapid diagnosis of a functional movement disorder is helpful, as psychological treatment can then be started. A video-EEG recording might be used as a diagnostic test in those with convulsions. Suppose a seizure-like event is captured, and the EEG stays relatively normal. In that case, a diagnosis of psychogenic nonepileptic attacks (also known as psychogenic nonepileptic seizures, pseudoseizures, or functional dissociative seizures) might be made.[45] This diagnosis makes an impact on the course of treatment. Once the diagnosis is made, medical testing is often reduced. Unnecessary medical testing may worsen matters, as the affected person may continue to believe that their symptoms are due to a medical and not a psychological condition.[46] The parents may occasionally seek alternative treatments, including medicinal supplements, antibiotics, or immunosuppressants, such as steroids or intravenous immunoglobulin. These treatments are expensive, have limited proven benefits, and can have serious side effects. Formal neuropsychological testing may help discover frequent co-occurring disorders, such as anxiety, depression, or post-traumatic stress disorder, that perhaps evaded early detection. A social worker can help discover school-based issues such as bullying. Sometimes a specific traumatic event can be found. Psychological evaluation, cognitive behavioral therapy, and counseling are the mainstay of treatment and may lead to symptom relief.[46] When combined with specific medications that target the associated psychological disturbance, psychiatric care can bring about a more rapid recovery.

Nonepileptic attacks

A 17-year-old girl began having intermittent episodes where she would thrash her arms and legs back and forth and would often hit or bump into objects. The events became more frequent and severe. She began to stumble around before falling to the floor. When help arrived, she appeared unconscious but awoke spontaneously and at once recognized the people around her. She seemed oriented and was not tired or confused. She was taken to her local emergency room several times. Brain imaging and EEG were normal. The events persisted. A continuous EEG with video monitoring was ordered. During the test, a similar convulsion occurred, but the EEG remained normal. She was diagnosed with psychogenic nonepileptic attacks and was referred to a psychologist and counselor for evaluation and cognitive behavioral therapy.

Tics rarely look like seizures, but this possibility might be considered and explored by a clinician when the movement first begins. A seizure is characterized by a rapid onset of abnormal behavior and movements (convulsion) caused by unregulated and chaotic brain activity. Tics and seizures are paroxysmal movements, as they tend to come and go, and they both may worsen with stress. Tics can appear seizure-like if the actions become persistent and rhythmic. While both seizures and tics can involve movements of the face, seizures can often be excluded by inspection. Consciousness requires at least one side of the brain to function normally. Therefore, seizures are unlikely if the child is awake and alert while both sides of the body are moving abnormally. However, it may be difficult for the clinician to know what is happening if the person does not show the movements in the office or if a video of the movements is unavailable. Therefore, clinicians may decide to order an EEG.

The results of an EEG will not show the doctor whether their patient had a seizure in the past, but it can help to determine whether there is a risk of seizures occurring in the future. EEG results can also be confusing, however, as many children with an abnormal EEG will never have a seizure.[47] Furthermore, persons with epilepsy can have normal EEGs in between seizures.[47] Capturing the movements while the EEG is running is very useful, as it can allow one to exclude the possibility of epileptic seizures definitively. However, EEG monitoring is generally unnecessary for persons with tics, as the diagnosis can often be made by studying the movements.

Some clinicians are uncomfortable diagnosing tics and will obtain an EEG just to be sure that the movements are not seizures. From time to time the EEG is not normal, but the abnormality has nothing to do with the tics. This can be confusing to all parties and on occasion may lead to inappropriate assumptions, inaccurate diagnosis, and/or improper treatments. Of course, some children can develop both epilepsy and a tic disorder. The two are not thought to be related and generally need to be treated as separate disorders. As discussed in chapter 4, some medications for epilepsy can also help to reduce the burden of tics.

Transient motor tics with an abnormal EEG

An 8-year-old girl developed intermittent eye-blinking and nose-scrunching movements. She was diagnosed with tics by her pediatrician and was referred to a neurologist for further evaluation. The neurologist ordered a brain MRI and performed an EEG. The MRI was normal, but the EEG was not. The EEG showed abnormal spike activity that could potentially lead to a seizure. No medications were given since the girl had never had a seizure. She was sent to a movement disorders clinic for a second opinion. It was decided that the movements were not consistent with a seizure, and no medications were started. The tics soon stopped. She was diagnosed with transient motor tics and an abnormal EEG. A repeat EEG was done a year later, and the results were normal.

Certain neurological diseases can cause tic-like movements of the face. Hemifacial spasm is a rare disorder where muscles on one side of the face twitch involuntarily.[48] Unlike tics, the movements only occur on one side of the face and do not change in character over time. The eye closes rapidly while the eyebrow moves upward. Sometimes the twitch spreads to other parts on the same side of the face, but only one side is affected. Hemifacial spasm is, therefore, quite unlike motor tics. Tics produce movements on both sides of the face or move sequentially from one side to the other. Tics can also differ from blepharospasm, a focal dystonia characterized by both eyes' forceful and prolonged closure.[49]

Wilson disease is a rare metabolic condition of copper storage.[50] Motor tics can be present in persons with Wilson disease,[51] but other symptoms, such as dystonia, are usually present as well. Dystonia is characterized by an involuntary muscle contraction that can slow repetitive movements and force the body into abnormal and sometimes painful positions. The muscle contractions may come and go or may be persistent. Sometimes the shaking or quivering resembles a tremor. Dystonia can look like a motor tic, but the dystonic movement is slower, with a sustained twisting or pulling motion. Wilson disease is a genetic disorder where copper is abnormally stored in the liver. Over time the liver reaches its storage limit, and copper begins to collect in other body parts, such as the kidneys, eyes, and brain. Those affected by Wilson disease are typically diagnosed when the pediatrician discovers liver dysfunction through routine laboratory studies. Screening for Wilson disease may be needed in adolescents who present with late-onset or atypical tics, along with other abnormal symptoms or signs on the neurological examination. Screening for the disease is done by blood and urine tests. Sometimes an eye examination and other testing are needed.

Sydenham's chorea is a rare movement disorder caused by the common bacterium *Streptococcus* behind "strep throat."[52] If left untreated, *Streptococcus* can sometimes produce various symptoms, including scarlet fever with a bright red skin rash, heart valve disease, and a movement disorder called chorea. Charcot and others in the late 1800s termed this movement disorder "true chorea," distinguishing it from tics and other movement disorders that produced similar symptoms. The disease is much less common now that antibiotics are available and used for strep throat. Chorea caused by *Streptococcus* is characterized by brief, irregular muscle contractions that are repetitive but not rhythmic. The arms, legs, and torso movements flow from one limb to another. Deciding whether the abnormal movements are due to tics or chorea can be challenging early in the illness. Unlike tics, children with chorea are aware of the movements and may sit on their hands to prevent them from moving. Suppressing the movements is nearly impossible, and there is no urge. Fortunately, Sydenham's chorea is generally a self-limited condition that resolves over several months. Medications are sometimes used to help dampen the movements if they become problematic.[53]

Over the years, clinicians and scientists have considered whether a tic disorder might be caused by the body's response to an infection.

Pediatric autoimmune neuropsychiatric disorders associated with streptococcal infections (PANDAS) is a proposed disorder whereby *Streptococcus* might cause obsessive-compulsive behaviors, tics, and/or other conditions.[54] The proposed mechanism for PANDAS is similar to that for Sydenham's chorea. In Sydenham's chorea, the immune system creates antibodies that target the streptococcal bacteria, as it should. However, these antibodies also target brain cells with similar proteins on their surface. Some physicians refer to this process as "molecular mimicry" or an "innocent bystander" reaction. Antibodies directed against the bacteria may specifically attack cells in the basal ganglia, which then do not work as they should. Unlike Sydenham's chorea, the immune system response that has been proposed to cause PANDAS does not apparently attack the heart and other body organs. Despite first being proposed in 1998, a link between streptococcal infection and the onset or worsening of a tic disorder has never been proven.[55] A review by Schrag and colleagues in 2022 showed that there was no clear association between group A streptococcal infection and the onset of tics.[55]

PANDAS?

A 5-year-old boy suddenly developed obsessive and compulsive thoughts and behaviors. He needed to open and close doors and turn on and off lights a certain number of times. He did not seem happy about these new behaviors, and they persisted at school and at home. He was seen by his pediatrician, who also noted the behaviors. The boy's examination was normal, except for a red and sore throat. A test for *Streptococcus* was positive, and he was treated with an antibiotic. His obsessive and compulsive movements declined over three weeks. When seen a month later by a neurologist, his examination was normal. No treatment was provided. The behaviors never returned, and he never developed tics.

Other similar autoimmune diseases called childhood acute neuropsychiatric symptoms (CANS), or pediatric acute-onset neuropsychiatric syndrome (PANS), have been proposed. It has been hypothesized that these disorders may be caused by an immune response initially directed toward a virus. Other proposed triggers that may lead to CANS or PANS include the "atypical" bacteria *Mycoplasma*, which causes pneumonia, and *Borrelia burgdorferi* acquired from a tick bite, which causes Lyme disease.[56] The main clinical components of these proposed disorders include abrupt onset of obsessive-compulsive symptoms and/or severe eating restrictions and concomitant cognitive, behavioral, or neurological symptoms.[57] Tics are not part of the core definition of PANS.[58] The proposed PANDAS, CANS, and PANS disorders are quite controversial, as there are no available confirmatory laboratory tests or specified treatments. There are several good review articles on the topic.[55,59–61]

Huntington's disease is a rare and incurable condition that runs in families.[62] It is a dominant genetic disorder. Generally, a grandparent or parent has been diagnosed with the disease before the child develops symptoms. Similar to Sydenham's chorea (see above), there are flowing movements of the extremities and torso. Unlike Sydenham's chorea, the chorea movements generally start in adulthood and inevitably worsen over time. Cognitive dysfunction, abnormal behaviors, and seizures often precede movement disorder when the disease begins in childhood.[63] Patient and family history can help exclude this disease, and genetic testing is not generally needed for persons with typical tics.

CHAPTER 4

Treatment and
Care

The diagnosis of tic disorder can be made by a pediatrician or a family practice provider. However, consultation with a specialist might be needed, especially when the diagnosis is unclear or the movements and sounds are complex. A second opinion by a neurologist, a psychologist, or a psychiatrist may be reasonable. The specialist might be someone who has considerable experience evaluating and treating someone with a tic disorder. The types of specialists who treat tics vary throughout the United States. In some regions, psychiatrists are comfortable making the diagnosis of tics and are able to treat both the tics and any co-occurring conditions. In other regions, neurologists make the diagnosis and provide the treatment, although they may not also manage the co-occurring conditions.

Should a Person with a Tic Disorder See a Neurologist, a Psychologist, a Therapist, or a Psychiatrist?

So, what is the difference between these medical specialists? A neurologist would see someone who might have an injury to the nervous system. A neurologist examines how the brain controls body function, such as movements and speech. Abnormal brain function might be suspected by the patient's history, physical and neurological examination findings, and abnormalities discovered on medical testing. The neurologist will perform a complete physical and neurological examination and may order tests if a problem is found. People with tics are expected to have a normal neurological examination. Perhaps surprising to parents, the person with tics may suppress their movements when they are visiting with the clinician in the examining room. If everything is expected to be normal, why does the pediatrician or primary care provider bother to send their patient to a neurologist? First of all, the clinician wants to exclude something "organic." This is an old term used to describe a brain problem that might be found on a neurological examination or a particular test.

Someone with a "nonorganic" disorder, characterized by abnormal thoughts and behaviors, might best be seen by a psychologist. A psychologist examines people's thoughts, emotions, and behaviors and can discover the most pertinent aspects of the person's disorder through interviews and formal assessment.

A therapist can be beneficial when people talk through their problems. A therapist is also essential when a type of behavioral therapy is recommended. As tics can be changed using behavioral approaches, a therapist nicely complements the medical team.

Input from a psychiatrist is helpful when medications might be needed to help control the psychological symptoms of a co-occurring condition. A multidisciplinary approach is helpful when tics occur with psychological conditions such as anxiety, obsessive-compulsive disorder (OCD), and/or attention-deficit/hyperactivity disorder (ADHD). The multidisciplinary approach is a coordinated effort by a medical team that may include a neurologist, psychologist, therapist, social worker, nurse, and psychiatrist.

How Can a Neuropsychologist and a Social Worker Help a Person with a Tic Disorder?

Neuropsychology is the study of how the brain affects the way people think and behave. Neuropsychologists help neurologists and psychologists assess the cause of their patients' behaviors. They aid with formulating correct diagnoses and help clinicians understand how neurological problems affect their patients' thinking skills and behavior. It is possible that the neuropsychologist will find a problem or disorder that the neurologist or psychologist was not actively considering. When details about the child's behavior are missing, the clinician might not consider some diagnoses. Therefore, for certain patients the neuropsychologist should be considered a necessary part of the health care team.

A complete neuropsychological assessment requires gathering and analyzing information about the child's education and physical, social, and psychological development. The neuropsychologist will collect the parent's observations of their child's motor skills, language acquisition, and social skills. The neuropsychologist then directly examines the child's ability to write, draw, speak, and think. A standardized assessment is used, as it is a reliable tool. Two of the most common tests include the Halstead-Reitan Neuropsychological Test Battery (which consists of the revised Wechsler Intelligence Scale for Children) and the Luria-Nebraska Neuropsychological Battery. Other standardized tests are sometimes used. The choice of test depends on the child's age and other factors. The neuropsychology assessment may take one to two days. A lengthy report is then generated, which summarizes the observations and supplies a set of scores that help to discover the child's strengths and weaknesses. Recommendations are often provided.

The neuropsychology report benefits parents and older patients who can better understand the problems, why specific behavioral interventions are needed, and what to expect in the future. Testing can be repeated periodically to determine whether the interventions have improved the person's symptoms. If a neuropsychological evaluation is obtained, the parents or patient should seriously consider sharing the report with their doctors, teachers, therapists, and advisors.

Parents and patients are understandably concerned about privacy. They may hesitate to share the neuropsychologist's report with anyone. The neuropsychology assessment may be most helpful if shared with the child's teacher. The report will highlight both the child's strengths and their shortcomings. While efforts are made to improve on any identified deficits, the parent and teacher can use the child's identified strengths to keep the child engaged and enhance their psychological well-being. While certain remedial activities will be needed to improve the child's weaknesses and abnormal behaviors, allowing the child to highlight their strengths in class can facilitate a cheerful disposition. Positive feedback will only encourage the child to improve their performance in other areas. The neuropsychology report will also help teachers serve children with learning disabilities more effectively. A child who has neurologically related disabilities may be helped by using strategies different from those used for other children.

There are limitations of a neuropsychological assessment. The test result depends on the training, skill, and experience of the expert performing the analysis. The evaluation is lengthy, and keeping the child engaged is necessary. Children with disabilities and psychological issues, as well as normal functioning children, can become distracted. A child who becomes fatigued will not do well in later parts of the assessment. The neuropsychologist must perform the evaluation in a proper setting that is engaging but not stressful. The child's cultural background and prior experiences may also change the test's outcome. For example, one child might say "flower" when shown a picture of a ceramic vase, while another might say "toothbrush holder." Understanding the child's cultural, social, and economic backgrounds can help to ensure that the evaluation is as correct as possible and that the results would be reproduced if the tests were administered by someone different in another setting. Performance scores included in the assessment are not perfect. It is essential to realize the neuropsychological assessment's limitations and understand that it is just one part of a complete evaluation. Parents and the health care team may occasionally disagree with the neuropsychologist's conclusions. There are multiple reasons why an assessment might need to be more accurate, and those reasons may be unrelated to the neuropsychologist's skill. When significant concerns about the validity of the evaluation arise, another evaluation should be performed when it is practical to do so.

Within the United States, neuropsychology testing is generally available in each school district. The Education for All Handicapped Children Act of 1975 and the Education of the Handicapped Act Amendments of 1986 require schools to find, screen, assess, and serve all disabled children who are 3 years old and older. This allows children to receive an education best suited to their needs. A benefit of a school-assigned neuropsychologist is that the evaluation will be performed at no charge. However, the patient and parent cannot choose who will perform the evaluation. A primary care provider or specialist can supply a good reference if a private assessment is desired. A social worker is also a good resource for identifying an appropriately trained and experienced neuropsychologist with a track record of excellence.

Social workers are an essential part of the patient's medical team. They help individuals, groups, and families prevent and cope with problems in their everyday lives. Social workers practice in various settings and focus their work on the community's needs. Social workers are employed in schools, clinics, and hospitals. They are essential to ensure the proper care of a person with a tic disorder. The social worker can function as a connection between the patient, clinician, teacher, and family. The social worker in the medical clinic can communicate with the social worker at school and help pass on important information that will assist with developing appropriate learning accommodations. They can advocate for the child and their family. They can also help with insurance, immigration, and legal issues. Social workers with special training can also supply cognitive behavioral therapy, including comprehensive behavioral intervention for tics (CBIT).

Is Treatment of a Tic Disorder Needed, and What Might Be Required?

Treatment may be helpful for persons with a tic disorder. Treatment is primarily determined by whether the tics negatively influence socialization, academics, or activities.[1,2] Once the diagnosis of a tic disorder is confirmed, several options are available. A period of observation and an effort to reduce stress are often the first step. Evaluation for co-occurring conditions that may provoke the tics is generally recommended.[3] If the tics persist and become troublesome, behavioral therapy and/or medications might become necessary.

What Treatment Options Are Available?

Oftentimes, the best treatment is to do nothing. A watchful waiting approach is often the best choice, especially for children with simple motor and/or vocal tics. Some children may develop transient tics that do not require any specific treatment. The tics might continue for a short time and then stop. Educating the patient, their parent, and their school team (if applicable) is often all that is needed. The clinician may discuss ways to reduce stress and social media use. The clinician may also ask questions to see whether the patient might have a co-occurring neuropsychological condition that often accompanies a tic disorder. A follow-up clinic visit, along with a discussion of possible treatments, may be considered later on if the tics persist or worsen.

Stress can undoubtedly have an impact on the frequency and severity of tics. Attempts to eliminate everyday stress are generally unsuccessful. Letting the child have a stress-free life with no household tasks and no need to do homework will result in a dysfunctional child. However, simple stress-reducing exercises and programs can be helpful, and both the child and their parents can take part. Relaxation training, hypnosis, psychotherapy, biofeedback, mindfulness-based practices, and self-monitoring have been used.[4] Such activities and treatments are not invasive, carry little risk, and may have long-lasting benefits. Most if not all of us could benefit from these activities, as they allow one to develop coping skills for stressful situations.

Social media can raise awareness for a particular disease and has helped create a sense of community among people with various disorders. However, there have been concerns about social media in the news and the medical literature. As discussed in chapter 3, teenage girls may have developed a functional movement disorder that mimics a severe motor and vocal tic disorder simply by watching "influencers" on social media platforms. Social media platforms allow children as young as 13 years to sign up. If the movements do not seem to be tics and seem more consistent with a functional movement disorder, the parents should consider restricting or removing social media platforms that may be affecting their child's health. The person with a tic disorder should consider that repeatedly watching a video of someone having their tic, or pretending to have a tic, will not help to reduce their own.

Children with a tic disorder should be evaluated for a co-occurring condition. These conditions include anxiety, OCD, and ADHD (see chap. 3). Tics and symptoms of these disorders occur together with significant frequency. Attempting to treat the tics without addressing these related conditions can be disappointing. For example, it is becoming clear that anxiety can provoke the premonitory urge and make the tic symptoms worse. Therefore, these co-occurring conditions may worsen the tics and, if left untreated, hinder other efforts that aim to reduce the tic burden.

Most of the time, parents will know if their child has challenges with anxiety, obsessions, or problems keeping attention. However, the symptoms of these disorders are sometimes difficult to detect. A child may be good at hiding their anxiety about certain situations. For example, their parent might be unaware of ongoing issues at school or challenges with certain social situations.

It is valuable to recognize obsessive-compulsive behaviors since they may mimic motor tics. A child who repetitively touches objects or makes movements or sounds in multiples of twos or threes may be showing obsessive-compulsive behaviors rather than tics. A diagnosis of an OCD rather than a tic disorder will change treatment recommendations.

Neuropsychology testing can help determine whether the child has a co-occurring condition. Some clinicians use the Vanderbilt ADHD Diagnostic Rating Scale for children aged 6–12 years.[5] The National Institute for Children's Health Quality's Vanderbilt Assessment Scales are available online. The parent and teacher answer questions about how well the child does with schoolwork and gets along with others. Besides screening for ADHD, the test also looks for other conditions such as conduct disorder, oppositional-defiant disorder, anxiety, and depression. The completed forms are then returned to the clinician for interpretation.

Other clinicians may use the Conners scale for ADHD assessment.[6,7] The Conners rating scale is a questionnaire that asks about things like behavior, work, schoolwork, and social life. There are different versions of the Conners rating scales. Parents and teachers usually fill out the scales for children. Older children and adults complete their own forms. Adults may ask their spouse, coworker, or close friend to complete one as well. Other useful tests for children with a suspected co-occurring condition include the Behavior Assessment System of Children and the Child Behavior Checklist/Teacher Report Form.[8,9]

Recommended treatments may include a referral to a school counselor or social worker, cognitive behavioral therapy, and/or medications. A social worker or counselor can be helpful since children may feel uncomfortable speaking with their parents about their inner thoughts and problems. As noted in the next section, cognitive behavioral therapy is often the first line of treatment for these conditions. However, medications may be needed if the symptoms prevent attendance in school or other activities.

Cognitive Behavioral Therapy

The purpose of cognitive behavioral therapy is to find unhealthy, negative beliefs and behaviors and replace them with healthy, adaptive ones. There are many different types of cognitive behavioral therapy.[10] Dialectical behavior therapy is a type of cognitive behavioral therapy that teaches skills to help someone manage distress, regulate emotions, and improve their relationships with others. Mindfulness-based therapy can help people recognize and understand the thoughts and actions of others. This can help reduce their anxiety and depression and improve their sense of well-being. Cognitive behavioral therapy is also helpful for treating adult ADHD. Here, the patient uses a combination of psychoeducation and distractibility delay, where one writes down distractions when they emerge rather than acting on the distraction.[11]

Habit reversal therapy, CBIT, and exposure-response prevention therapy are types of cognitive behavioral therapy that help to reduce the frequency of tics, even more so than medications.[3,4,12] Habit reversal therapy consists of (1) recognizing the premonitory urge that precedes the disruptive tic and (2) developing a competing volitional or willful response that is physically incompatible with the tic.[13] The new deliberate response to the urge may interrupt the reinforcement cycle between the urge and the tic. Habit reversal therapy is the primary therapeutic element of CBIT.

CBIT is considered by many to be a first-line therapy for older children with a tic disorder.[14] CBIT works on the premise that breaking the cycle between the urge and the tics can break up the habit.[15] Like cognitive behavioral therapy for bad habits, the intervention relies on habit recognition and substitution, yet it includes additional behavioral assessments and treatments. CBIT is helpful if the person with tics (1) recognizes the tic, (2) recognizes the premonitory urge that occurs before the tic, and (3) is motivated to get rid of the tic.

The CBIT approach includes the following measures:

- Recognizing the premonitory urge that precedes the disruptive tic.
- Developing a competing volitional or willful response that is physically incompatible with the tic.
- Psychoeducation.
- Function-based assessments and interventions.
- Behavioral incentives.

So how does CBIT work? When an urge is detected, the person replaces the tic with a new movement, but the new movement is entirely voluntary. For example, instead of letting the tic move the head to the right shoulder, the left hand is brought to the right shoulder. This competing response helps to quench the urge and replace the automatic tic with a purposeful movement. This competing response is sometimes called "tic blocking." The replacement movement conflicts with the tic and can stop the tic from happening.

Psychoeducation includes gathering information and discussing the diagnosis throughout the course of treatment. Function-based assessments and interventions find and address factors that worsen the tic such as teasing, classroom conditions, meeting new people, and challenging schedules. Behavioral incentives include rewards to help motivate the person with a tic disorder to take part in sessions and encourage practice at home. Patients also receive instruction in muscle relaxation and controlled breathing. This relaxation training can help reduce stress that is caused by the tic. It may also help the patient cope with excitement, anxiety, or other stressors that can worsen the tics.

The CBIT program consists of the following objectives:

- Training the person to be aware of their urge and their tic.
- Teaching the person to perform competing movements when they feel the premonitory urge to make a tic.
- Making lifestyle changes that can help reduce the tics.

The CBIT program can vary somewhat between therapists. During the first visit, the therapist may collect information, supply an overview of the program, and set expectations. If a decision is made to move forward, the program consists of up to eight weekly sessions. Up to three more refresher or booster sessions at various intervals may be needed or recommended. The length of treatment will depend on several individual factors, including patient participation and response. Oftentimes, the therapist will target and focus on the single most bothersome tic. The less intrusive tics may be addressed in later sessions. Sessions with younger children are completed jointly with a parent, while those for older adolescents might be performed individually, with parent consent. Some patients and therapists prefer face-to-face visits, while others favor remote sessions using an internet-based platform. The therapist may follow the child's progress and the effect of CBIT using a tic rating scale. This can supply an objective assessment as to whether CBIT has been helpful over the course of treatment. The Yale Global Tic Severity Scale is the most extensively used test.[16]

CBIT is only useful for some persons with tics. As mentioned previously, young children are often unaware of their tics and, therefore, are not interested in therapy for a problem that does not exist in their mind. Once the child becomes "self-aware," they may begin to recognize the problem and seek help. Like all therapies, CBIT needs a willing participant who will learn from their therapist and practice at home. CBIT is challenging, and it requires much effort by the patient to work. Older adolescents who have already developed a tic-blocking technique may not be interested in attending therapy, as it simply reminds them about their tics, which may increase the frequency of the movements.

Several clinical trials have proven the usefulness of CBIT.[3] The effect of CBIT is similar to that of medications.[17] In a recent clinical trial, 30 percent of patients who received 10 weeks of CBIT showed improvement in tic severity, compared to 14 percent of those who only received supportive therapy.[18] It is still to be determined whether continued benefits occur after treatment with medication. However, 87 percent of patients who received CBIT showed continued benefit six months after finishing their training. This might be a consideration when weighing the time required for multiple sessions of CBIT. Therefore, CBIT should be tried if the person with tics who feels the premonitory urge is motivated and a therapist with experience in CBIT is available.

The tics are treated with CBIT

An 11-year-old girl began making intermittent purring sounds like a cat. Her mother recalled that the girl had been blinking repetitively six years before. She had been seen by an eye specialist and an allergist, but the blinking stopped a few months after they had begun without intervention. As a new first-year student in high school, she seemed under stress, but she denied this when her parents inquired. The girl's neurological examination was normal, and she was diagnosed with a chronic motor and vocal tic disorder. She was referred to a counselor for stress reduction. Four weeks later the purring noises stopped but were replaced by repetitive head thrusting. As she could feel a need to make the movements and sounds, she was referred to a therapist for CBIT. Different tics developed, but she was able to control them by intermittently meeting with her therapist for a CBIT refresher session.

████ ████ ████ ████ ████ ████ ████ ████ ████ ████ ████ ████

Another psychological approach that has shown benefits for persons with tics in clinical trials is exposure-response prevention therapy.[4] Exposure-response prevention therapy is based on the idea that a conditioned response (tic) to a premonitory urge is strengthened by repetition. This may seem to imply that the longer the tics continue, the worse the urge and the more difficult it becomes for a person with tics to stop. However, there is not much evidence to support this assumption.[3] Exposure-response prevention therapy aims to interrupt this cycle by training persons with tics to tolerate the urge and suppress the tics for long periods. Of course, ignoring the urge is like going "cold turkey." This can be very difficult for children and adults, and strong support from their therapist, family, and friends is needed. Exposure-response prevention therapy is the first-line treatment for OCD.[19]

It is still unclear exactly how cognitive behavioral therapy, CBIT, or exposure-response therapy help to reduce tics. These techniques may theoretically help reprogram the function of brain circuits that develop and support habits. As in habit reversal therapy, which focuses on cues and movements, CBIT disconnects the urge from the tic. The premonitory urge may then eventually lessen over time. Both habit reversal therapy and exposure-response prevention therapy may substantially reduce tic severity. Both approaches have similar levels of success.[20]

What Do the Internet and Clinical Trials Have to Offer?
The internet is ripe with information. Some of it is useful, and a lot of it is not. The parent or patient with a tic disorder will likely go online to discover what they have and what can help. In this section, we will

outline the risks and benefits of using the internet to search for useful information and how one might navigate prior or ongoing clinical trials that may impact the person with a tic disorder.

Should someone consult with Dr. Google? Who is Dr. Google, and where did they get their degree? Nowhere and everywhere are both correct. A massive amount of information is available to read. Although a lot of information on the internet is correct, much of it is inaccurate. The *Telegraph* reported that up to 7 percent of Google's daily searches are health related. Over 70,000 searches per minute translate into over 1 billion searches on health-related topics each day.[21] Early predictions in 2013 suggested that there could be as much as 2,314 exabytes of health-related data by 2020. An exabyte is a vast number—add 16 zeros. A recent Google search posted 853,000,000 results for tic, 30,900,000 for a tic disorder, and 11,300,000 for Tourette's syndrome.

Which search results are the best ones to read? Suppose a parent was interested in spending hundreds or thousands of hours researching a tic disorder. Is it better to start at the beginning of the search result, in the middle, or at the end? Would it matter? People created search algorithms to organize the world's information. A recent report in the *Wall Street Journal* suggested that algorithms may favor big business.[22] The excited web searcher will soon find that articles provide the same brief description of a tic disorder, with a link so that you can make an appointment. One might start seeing scientific papers or reviews. Scientific articles may post the results of a clinical trial that tried to determine whether a tic disorder is related to another condition or whether a particular treatment works to reduce tics. It can be challenging to figure out whether the results of a clinical trial are pertinent for your child. Another issue is the large volume of unreliable information where people tell personal stories that may not apply to other people with a tic disorder and suggest treatments that are dangerous or have no scientific basis.

Do clinical trials help? Scientists who have worked in the field for years have realized that a lot of published data are preliminary, and the conclusions are controversial. The presence of controversial data does not mean that scientists are careless. The work is challenging, and each patient in a study is a bit different. For every scientific study that reports that one thing is related to another, there may be another study that shows that they are not. The results of a survey may be different if the experimental conditions change. Various brain problems may cause similar symptoms. Scientists need to repeat experiments so that the truth appears over time. By presenting data at national conferences, a consensus begins to appear. The nonscientist may seek the truth by reading scientific reports and reviews, but the details need to be more transparent for most of us to understand.

On occasion, the participants who took part in the study can have a different set of problems than the reader or the reader's child. Scientists try to tease out a subset of patients to study. For example, pooling together people who have the symptoms needed to diagnose Tourette's disorder allows the scientist to have a more focused group of study patients. However, study patients who met the diagnosis of Tourette's disorder may have an array of co-occurring conditions that might affect the research outcome. Replicating the result of a clinical trial is necessary to discover the truth.

Suppose a study shows that a particular medication helps more children with tics than a placebo. In that case, the scientist and the drug company conclude that the medicine is a reasonable choice for tics. But how does the scientist reach that conclusion? The scientist runs a particular statistical test. A "statistically significant" result means that there is a greater than 95 percent chance that the medication will help someone with that particular problem. Still, the amount of benefit will differ between people.

What is a placebo-controlled clinical trial? A placebo is anything that seems to be correct but is not. When a new medication is being evaluated, the scientist must exclude a "placebo effect." The act of simply taking a pill can have a positive effect on symptoms. The person believes that the medicine, no matter what is in it, will help the symptoms, and sometimes it does. Therefore, the result of a placebo often depends on the person's expectations. Suppose a person thinks that a medication might cause problems, such as drowsiness or irritability. In that case, there is a greater chance that these reactions will happen. Tics might be particularly vulnerable to placebo. As discussed in chapter 1, the neurochemical dopamine, which acts on areas of the brain to provide feelings of pleasure, satisfaction, and motivation, is thought to take part in developing and keeping habits. The amount of dopamine in the brain may increase when the person is exposed to a new situation, such as taking a new medication. Therefore, any new medicines might reduce tics owing to a placebo effect.

What is a randomized, double-blinded, placebo-controlled clinical trial? There are different types of clinical trials, and this type of trial may be the best. Study patients are randomly divided into two or more treatment groups. One group receives the test medication. Another group gets half the dose. A third group takes a medication-free pill called a placebo. Other approaches are used depending on the study. The trial is "double-blinded" when both the study participant and the clinician are unaware of the assigned treatment group. Neither the patient nor the clinician knows whether the patient is taking the medication or the placebo. At the end of the clinical trial, an outcome is decided, and the results are published. The study patient may never know whether they took the medication or the placebo. In addition, the study patient may not be able to keep taking the medication even if it seemed to help the symptoms. More clinical trials may need to be done before the medication is available at the pharmacy.

There are funding challenges for clinical trials and basic science. Clinical trials are time-consuming, and they cost a lot of money. The more complex and, therefore, more valid the trial, the more it costs to run. A clinical trial requires hundreds of hours and an enormous commitment by patients, physicians, assistants, statisticians, and administrators. Besides setting up the experiment, there are safety factors to consider. An institutional review board carefully considers the clinical trial to ensure that it is safe for the patients who enroll in the study. Frequent monitoring with office visits and tests is generally needed.

The costs for any clinical trial are tremendous, so a sponsor is necessary. Unfortunately, the funding for clinical trials and basic science experiments is low. The US government supplies funding for patient registries or outcome trials, and pharmaceutical companies promote and fund clinical trials for new medications. Foundations, such as the Tourette Association of America, offer small grants to investigators. Otherwise, funding comes from gifts made by the community or donors in the form of philanthropy. A lack of funding for clinical trials might explain why, for example, there are few data on using vitamins or minerals, such as magnesium, for a tic disorder. The lack of funding also impacts our ability to understand the neurological and genetic mechanisms that contribute to the development of a tic disorder. When a person with tics is reading about the result of a clinical trial, they need to determine whether the results are truly applicable to their situation. The trial's outcome may be exciting, but other medications might still be better. It is essential to discuss the clinical trial with their clinician.

What Medications Can Be Used for a Tic Disorder?

While treatment options like CBIT should be considered first, tics that impact the child's well-being, education, and out-of-school activities should be taken seriously, and medications can help.[23] Several prescription medications may help to improve tics, including antihypertensives, anticonvulsants, antipsychotics, and others (box 4.1).[24]

BOX 4.1

Medications Sometimes Used to Treat Tics

Medication	Type	Mechanism
Guanfacine (Tenex)	Antihypertensive	Activates the alpha-2 receptors
Clonidine (Catapres)	Antihypertensive	Activates the alpha-2 receptors
Topiramate (Topamax)	Anticonvulsant	Decreases excitation in the brain
Levetiracetam (Keppra)	Anticonvulsant	Decreases excitation in the brain
Baclofen	Muscle relaxant	Stimulates GABA-B receptors
Aripiprazole (Abilify)	Atypical antipsychotic	Blocks dopamine receptors
Risperidone (Risperdal)	Atypical antipsychotic	Blocks dopamine receptors
Haloperidol (Haldol)	Antipsychotic	Blocks dopamine receptors
Pimozide (Orap)	Antipsychotic	Blocks dopamine receptors
Tetrabenazine (Xenazine)	VMAT inhibitor	Reduces dopamine in the brain
Diphenhydramine (Benadryl)	Antihistamine	Provides mild sedation (likely mechanism)

The medications may help reduce the number and frequency of tics by changing brain receptors or the amount of a specific neurotransmitter released into the brain.[25] All of these medications were created to treat other diseases but were later found to be helpful for tics. When a medication designed for one disorder is found to be beneficial for another, it is called a "repurposed medication." Tics can be reduced when small doses of these repurposed medications are used. The amount of a repurposed medication is generally much lower than the dose used for the medication's primary purpose. Lowering the dose of medication helps to avoid any potential unwanted effects. For example, guanfacine was made to treat high blood pressure (hypertension). A small amount of guanfacine may improve tics without lowering blood pressure. Sometimes an antipsychotic medication is used, not because a child is psychotic but because the medication has been shown to help reduce tics.

None of the available medications will cure the tic disorder. The treatment goal of these medications is to reduce tics to the point that they are no longer interfering with normal function or causing distress. Different drugs may need to be tried, as medications may work for one person but not another. However, a careful examination of the benefits and risks of each medication is always needed. All of the medicines that are available to treat tics have potential side effects. This does not mean that the treatment will cause side effects.

The antipsychotic medications haloperidol, pimozide, and aripiprazole are the only medications approved for treating tics by the US Food and Drug Administration (FDA).[3,26] However, clinicians may use repurposed "off-label" (i.e., not approved by the FDA for treatment of tics) medications, as they may be better tolerated and have fewer potential side effects. The medications more often used for tics are guanfacine and clonidine.[26] These medications are FDA approved for treating ADHD symptoms, so they can be helpful in children with both tics and ADHD. Guanfacine and clonidine were initially designed for the treatment of high blood pressure. Since they can occasionally cause dizziness and mild sedation, they are generally given at bedtime. A once-a-day dose at bedtime may be enough. Guanfacine and clonidine last about 12–17 hours, so twice-daily dosing is sometimes needed. If breakthrough tics occur when the child returns home from school, a second, perhaps smaller dose of guanfacine can be given in the afternoon. Extended-release forms are available, but they can be more expensive, and they may have a greater chance of causing heart rhythm abnormalities.[26] Clonidine is also available as a transdermal (skin) patch that has been shown to reduce tic burden.[27] It is an attractive alternative to oral clonidine treatment for some people, as it may reduce sedation, due to more consistent blood levels, and eliminate the need to take several doses of medication each day.[28] The decision to use a medication should be discussed with the patient's clinician. The type of medication, as well as the dose and timing, will need to be carefully considered. It is important to know that there is no evidence that medical treatment for a tic disorder is more effective the earlier it is started.[3]

Parents need to be patient when a medication is just started. "Start at a low dose and go slow" is the idea, so medication increases may be needed before an improvement is seen. Further, since tics may come and go over time, it is sometimes difficult to decide whether a medication supplies relief in the first few weeks or months of treatment. In other words, a drug will work well if it is started when the tic frequency is at a peak, as the tics were destined to improve whether the medication was used or not. Suppose the tics are infrequent when a medication is started. In that case, the natural rise in tic frequency might be mistakenly blamed on the medication. Therefore, it is essential for the parent to be patient and to closely follow the instructions of the child's clinician. Similarly, if a decision is made to stop the medication, the doctor may recommend a plan to slowly taper the dose over several weeks.

Medications called anticonvulsants, initially developed to control seizures, may also be helpful for tic disorders. Topiramate has been shown to improve motor tics in several clinical trials.[29-31] While the drug may have potential side effects such as sedation, appetite suppression, or word-finding difficulties, these may not occur at the low doses typically used for tics. Low-dose topiramate is also quite useful for migraine headaches, another "paroxysmal" disorder where symptoms come and go. Another anticonvulsant medication called levetiracetam (Keppra) may help reduce tics.[32] Selective serotonin reuptake inhibitors (SSRIs) might also be effective for tics, as they can help with some of the co-occurring conditions. SSRIs work best for persons with tics who also have anxiety, OCD, or depression.[33] Botulinum toxin may be helpful for highly focal tics in older adolescents and adults.[34] Baclofen, a GABA-B receptor stimulator (agonist), may also be beneficial.[35]

Antipsychotics, also known as neuroleptics or major tranquilizers, block dopamine receptors in the brain. Their ability to reduce tics led to modern theories about the brain pathways that might underly the disorder. The three most studied antipsychotics are haloperidol, pimozide, and risperidone.[36-38] Aripiprazole (Abilify) is the most widely used medication for those diagnosed with Tourette's disorder.[39] While many antipsychotics are available, recent studies have failed to show that one of these medications is superior to the others.[40,41] The drugs are quite potent, and they will likely reduce the tics. However, these antipsychotic drugs may also have a higher incidence of side effects, such as weight gain, sedation, anxiety, and heart rhythm changes. On occasion, antipsychotics can cause another movement disorder called tardive dyskinesia.[23] These and other potential side effects should be discussed with the child's clinician. Of course, the benefits of the medication should be considered alongside the potential risks.

Some persons may develop a tic storm, an episode of severe and unrelenting tics that stops as abruptly as it began. In some cases, these tic storms occur in the setting of a long period of tic suppression. Diphenhydramine (Benadryl) supplied once, at a typical dose used for allergies, can be very effective in calming these storms, perhaps by promoting a degree of sedation. The use of Benadryl for a tic storm should be discussed with the child's clinician.

Deep brain stimulation may be considered in those persons with severe and intractable motor and vocal tic disorder.[13] A neurosurgeon permanently places a thin metal electrode into a part of the brain's basal ganglia or thalamus. Small amounts of current are delivered to stimulate or block brain circuits. Deep brain stimulation is often used in persons with Parkinson's disease, and it appears safe and effective for persons with Tourette's disorder.[42] As some may experience acute adverse effects, several medications should have failed for these patients before considering deep brain stimulation. The device should only be offered at experienced centers after an evaluation by a multidisciplinary team.[43] A local ethics committee or institutional review board should be consulted when considering deep brain stimulation for people younger than 18 years of age.[43]

Several nonconventional therapies have been proposed for people with a tic disorder, but there is not enough evidence to support their use.[3] These therapies include medical marijuana, acupuncture, and vitamins. The use of medical marijuana (cannabis) for tic disorder is still under investigation.[44] Medical marijuana has two chemicals: delta-9-tetrahydrocannabinol (THC) and cannabidiol (CBD). These chemicals are currently used to treat people with a tic disorder in several countries, including Canada, Israel, and Germany. There are isolated reports that medical marijuana is helpful, while others have reported side effects or no help. The Tourette Association of America says that there are insufficient data to support the use of CBD without adding THC.[44] THC is considered a mind-altering drug, and the main effect of the drug might be problematic, especially for a developing child.

Compared to THC, CBD is better tolerated, and it seems to be an effective medication for anxiety or OCD, at least during the initial stages of treatment.[45] Since anxiety and OCD are known to increase the frequency and severity of tics, CBD may be a potential treatment, but additional research is needed.[45] One particular CBD medication called Epidiolex was approved for the treatment of rare forms of epilepsy.[44] Epidiolex may not be covered by insurance if prescribed for treating other disorders, such as tics. CBD oil is available in local dispensaries but is unregulated by the FDA. CBD's quality, potency, and consistency may vary from one batch to the next. The unmeasured and unpredictable amount of CBD provided by a CBD dispensary makes it difficult for clinicians to recommend a dose. CBD treatment should be avoided in children and adolescents because of the lack of data and the association with negative long-term cognitive effects.[3,26]

Medical marijuana has both THC and CBD. The FDA does not currently regulate it, and its use is not currently authorized under federal law. However, it may be available in different states. Marijuana is still listed as an FDA schedule 1 drug, preventing large-scale research studies from being conducted in the United States. There is little evidence that THC reduces tics and abundant evidence that it impairs cognitive function in children and adolescents.[3,46] Supplying unproven treatments to children for tics is not advisable unless it is under the supervision of the child's clinician.

Acupuncture is a branch of traditional Chinese medicine that has been used for thousands of years. Acupuncture involves placing fine needles into certain acupoints that were defined by traditional Chinese medicine theory. A literature review performed in 2016 suggested that acupuncture may be an effective secondary therapy that could improve the outcome of standard medical treatments that are typically used for a tic disorder.[47] However, evidence that acupuncture is helpful is limited, and some reports that claim that acupuncture reduces tic symptoms may be biased.[47]

Vitamins and supplements have been shown to alleviate migraine headaches. However, there are currently no good studies with evidence for the benefit of vitamins and supplements in treating patients with a tic disorder. The use of vitamin D3, vitamin B6, and magnesium has been proposed, but more investigations are needed. Similarly, some parents try dietary changes, but due to a lack of financial resources, clinical trials to determine whether such diets are helpful have yet to be conducted.

A parent's preference or predisposition may sometimes impact the decision to medicate a child with a tic disorder. Though parents listen closely to the clinician's advice, sometimes they come into the office with prejudice about whether they want to leave with a medication prescription. Parents of a child with tics may have read about the transient nature of the disorder and that the tics may soon resolve on their own. They come to the clinician for assurance that their understanding of the disorder is correct and that there is nothing else to fear. Most parents are happy to hear that only observation is needed. Others have decided that medications are now needed, as the tics are causing discomfort or interfering with the child's life.

A minority of parents display fear of medications and will refuse to treat their child with medication no matter how severe the tics might be. The preference to not use drugs may come from the parents' experiences with clinicians and drugs that are unrelated to their child's problem. Another subset of parents may refuse to leave the office without a prescription. They want something to show for their efforts and want to help their child. Clinicians must understand the opinion and position of the parent early in the discussion. The patient should be included in the conversation, as they may have a different view. This helps to pave the way for a proper discussion about treatment benefits and risks. An agreement between the clinician, the parent, and the patient is essential for safety and compliance reasons. It is not a good idea for the clinician to prescribe for someone who will not take the medication. Alternatively, it is a problem when the clinician thinks that a prescription is needed, but the patient or their parent refuses. It can also be a problem when the parent wants a medication that is not needed. These situations require that the clinician carefully listen to the reasons behind the parent's or patient's position. Sometimes the clinician will need to send the patient to another clinician for a second opinion. Coming to a mutually agreeable decision with proper follow-up or referral to another clinician is sometimes the best approach. It is wise for the parent and patient to listen closely to the clinician's reasons in defense of their position. While treating tics is often unnecessary, behavioral approaches or medications are sometimes needed when the tics negatively affect the child.

Those parents or patients who are considering medications for a tic disorder might review the American Academy of Neurology's Practice Guideline Recommendations Summary.[3] More information about ongoing clinical trials for a tic disorder and Tourette's disorder is available at clinicaltrials.gov.

How Do Therapies and Medications Help to Reduce the Burden of Tics?

Learned behaviors and movements are thought to be programmed by brain cells within deeper portions of the brain called the basal ganglia.[48] Learning occurs when a repeated action changes the way cells communicate with each other. These changes in cell communication are not permanent. They cannot be erased, but they can theoretically be changed again by learning a new movement that substitutes for the old one. Alternatively, certain medications can be used to redesign the communication between cells.[49,50] Like painting over a picture, the underlying drawing stays, but it becomes modified by the new pigment.

Changes in brain circuitry may help explain why cognitive behavioral therapies can be beneficial. Once a person with a bad habit recognizes both the cue and the abnormal behavior, a new routine can be used to curb the premonitory cue. Similarly, once the person with tics recognizes the urge and the tic, a new purposeful or volitional movement is placed directly between the urge and the tic. This new movement then acts to block the tic. Since the brain begins to believe that the tic occurred, the urge is satisfied. Like any newly learned task, purposeful movement may theoretically act to reprogram the responsible brain circuit, and the habit or tic may be extinguished.

While a change in the number or sensitivity of brain receptors may explain features of brain plasticity, other changes in brain chemistry can and do occur.[2] Subtler changes occur within a learning brain, and the extent of these changes depends on different genetic and environmental factors. In this way, the tendency to develop habits varies widely across the population. This variability may be caused by differences in people's genes or environment.[51] The same might be true for tics. All of us might be at risk of developing tics, but certain people might be more susceptible than others. The cause of this susceptibility is still unclear.

CHAPTER 5

Support for the Child at School, Home, and Beyond

Many persons with a tic disorder will have mild and intermittent movements that do not affect their ability to socialize, learn, or regulate emotions. Others may have challenges in school and may have difficulties relating to friends, other students, or even family members. Issues related to the tics may develop. Movements and noises can be distracting for others and can be embarrassing for the person with tics. The presence of a co-occurring psychological condition can amplify these issues, and other problems might develop. In this chapter, we will discuss interventions at school and at home that can make a big impact on the person's well-being and help them succeed in the classroom.

School Plans and Accommodations for a Student with a Tic Disorder

Persons with mild and intermittent tics will likely not need any individualized plans for school. However, those with obtrusive tics and/or symptoms of a co-occurring condition such as anxiety, obsessive-compulsive disorder (OCD), or attention-deficit/hyperactivity disorder (ADHD), or those with a learning disability, may require more support from their teachers and school to compete fairly in the classroom.

Accommodations and modifications may be established through a 504 plan. If special education is necessary, an Individualized Education Plan (IEP) may be better. A 504 plan is developed to ensure that a student with an illness or a disability has equal access to education. In contrast, an IEP is designed to meet a student's unique needs. With the help of school officials, the parent must decide whether an IEP is necessary or whether a 504 plan is sufficient. An IEP requires more support for the student and increases the school's staffing needs.[1]

A 504 plan is a formal plan that schools develop to supply support for children who have special needs or a disability. The plan finds particular needs and identifies solutions that will help the child succeed at school. The plan also helps to prevent discrimination. The 504 plan is covered under Section 504 of the Rehabilitation Act, a civil rights law.[2] The 504 plan provides accommodations that the student may need to compete fairly in the classroom; it alters how a child will learn but does not alter what a child is expected to know. The plan might include extended time for tests, the ability to leave the classroom for short breaks, or a seat at the front. Accommodations may include study skill classes, time to speak with a school psychologist or social worker, or various treatments such as occupational, speech, and physical therapy. A 504 plan may occasionally include a modification. Unlike an accommodation that may be obtained under an IEP, a modification does alter what a student is expected to learn. Students may get fewer homework assignments or may be graded in a different way than others in the class. A 504 plan is not part of a special education plan. Those who need special education will require an IEP.

An IEP is a program that lays out a map of special education instruction, supports, and services that a child may need to make progress and thrive in school. It is developed to ensure that a child aged 3 years and older with an identified disability attending a primary or secondary educational institution or charter school receives specialized instruction and needed services. Most private schools do not offer IEPs. Still, students in a private school may be able to get special education through what is known as an Individual Service Plan. The IEPs are covered under the Disabilities in Education Act. There are no IEPs in college, but eligible students may apply for accommodations through their college disability service.

An IEP should be considered if the student needs specific support for anxiety, disorganization, sensory processing, or social skill deficits. The IEP is developed with the child by specialists, family members, or advocates. The IEP often includes the child in the general school curriculum and then adds necessary educational accommodations to help the child succeed. The IEP supplies measurable goals and aims for the child's education and includes all related services for which the child qualifies. Most children with an IEP remain in the same classroom as their peers. Testing performed by the child's school initially prepares the child for special education. The parents can also request outside testing, but the school decides eligibility.

What should be included in a 504 plan or IEP for children with tics? The content of a plan largely depends on the child's needs. These plans should be developed with the help of the school. The school does not have to write the plans, but most do. The school will need to review any pertinent clinicians' notes and may request more information from the child's medical team. An excellent guide for classroom strategies and techniques for children with a tic disorder and a co-occurring condition has been developed by the Tourette Association of America.[3]

The educational plan for those with a tic disorder should consider the following items, depending on the student's symptoms and needs:

- Provide a separate test location with extended time limits.
- Educate students in the class about tic disorder.

- Supply a safe place where the student can go to release their tics.
- Allow the student short breaks from the classroom.
- Help the student think of different ways to express their tics.
- Brainstorm other potential solutions with the student.

The plan for students with a tic disorder and anxiety might also include the following accommodations, depending on the student's symptoms and needs:

- Allow a transition time between activities.
- Allow extended testing time and/or an alternative testing environment.
- Allow the student to leave the classroom a few minutes early to avoid crowded hallways.
- Have a teacher aide nearby in the cafeteria to prevent confrontations. An alternative eating site with a friend may be ideal.
- Assign a seat in the front of the school bus and educate the bus driver.
- Develop and support strategies that diminish anxiety through self-help techniques.
- Consider an environment that will support the student.
- Show the student that their needs will be supported with respect.

A student with a tic disorder can have obsessive-compulsive behaviors, which can be overwhelming and result in increased stress, anxiety, and sometimes anger. Obsessions and compulsions can take different forms, so it can be challenging to supply general strategies.

Accommodations for students with a tic disorder and obsessive-compulsive behaviors might also include the following, depending on the student's symptoms and needs:

- An audiobook might be used by a student who is obsessed with counting words in every line.
- Hand sanitizer might be provided for a student with a germ obsession.
- A mechanical pencil could be used by a student who needs a perfectly sharpened pencil to write.
- A computer or tablet could be provided to a student with a writing obsession.
- A student with organizational difficulties may be helped by making lists.

A student with a tic disorder may have challenges maintaining attention. These students may also seem to move about constantly, fidget, tap, or talk at inappropriate times. The plan for students with tics and ADHD may also include the following, depending on the student's symptoms and needs:

- Offer or supply preferential seating in the classroom. A seat at the front and off to one side of the class, where the teacher can help the student to stay on task, may be ideal. The center front seat may be embarrassing for someone with tics.
- Allow for some freedom of movement, such as a quick trip to the bathroom or water fountain.
- Supply a quiet place to work in the classroom. Earphones with music or earplugs might help block out distractions. The teacher might establish a hand gesture or signal as a reminder for the student to refocus, get back on task, or communicate a need.

- Break down long-range assignments and projects into shorter, more manageable parts.
- Dispense one assignment at a time rather than all assignments at once.
- Supply a daily assignment sheet. The sheet should be completed by the student and verified by the teacher for accuracy. The parent should then check to make sure that all the work was completed.
- Help with homework prioritizing and management.
- Establish a line of communication between the teacher and an adult at home.
- A resource or consultant teacher should be considered, as a part of the team, to help with workload management and to help other teachers with reasonable expectations for the student. This person teaches lifelong strategies for organization and time management.

The educational plan for students with a tic disorder and language deficits might include the following, depending on the student's symptoms and needs:

- Provide a tablet, computer, and/or scribe as an accommodation.
- Avoid overpenalizing students for poor handwriting and/or spelling errors.
- Supply alternatives for written tests or assignments.
- Consider allowing oral, taped, or typed answers.
- Provide a highlighter to mark multiple-choice answers.
- Encourage the use of a computer spell check and/or grammar check.
- Supply a copy of the class notes rather than asking the student to copy them.

- Verify all homework assignments.
- Waive time limits on tests or allow extra time to reduce stress and anxiety.
- Condense or reduce assignments when possible.
- Supply graph paper to help line up math problems.

A person with a tic disorder may also have challenges managing sensory input. Students with tics can have difficulty transitioning from one activity to another because of sudden and unexpected sensory stimulation. Loudness, brightness, smells, touch, and other sensations are amplified in someone with sensory hypersensitivity. Some students with tics may have low sensitivity to stimulation. Low sensitivity to stimulation can make a student crave sensory stimulation that could lead to the need for loud and even harsh behavior, physical actions, and reactions. Students can have particular sensory needs, and an individualized sensory plan can be critical to the student's success. A plan for children with tics and a sensory processing disorder may include the following, depending on the child's needs:

- Minimize, as able, overstimulation in crowded hallways, cafeterias, school buses, playgrounds, and other unstructured settings.
- Provide the student with strategies to cope with an overstimulating environment.
- Encourage student participation with a school counselor or specialist.

Developing appropriate learning strategies and accommodations for a child requires a team effort. It is essential to first assess the nature of the child's symptoms and then brainstorm possible solutions with the child, teacher, and members of the medical team. It is important for parents to realize that schools can be understaffed and resources are often limited. It may take some creativity to come up with the best approach. The parent, student, and teacher should periodically reassess the student's accommodations to determine whether they need to be changed. Successful strategies to help the student may evolve over time. In certain instances, students may receive specific clinical therapies outside the school, such as comprehensive behavioral intervention for tics (CBIT). Such treatments may require different classroom approaches.

Guidance for Parents and Teachers

A pediatrician or other clinician can make a diagnosis of a tic disorder. Some children may have already been diagnosed with a different psychological condition. Still, there may be unanswered questions, persistent concerns, fear of treatments, and a thirst for knowledge. Parents are concerned about their child's social life and potential bullying at school. Parents may have taken to the internet to find answers, only to be confronted with a lifetime of reading. Scientific publications focus on very specific issues, and much of the information seems to be conflicting. The previous chapters focused on the frequency, cause, and treatment of a tic disorder. This section discusses some of the more common topics that interest parents.

My child has a tic disorder. Does this mean that they will develop yet another psychological problem? As discussed in chapter 3, the main co-occurring conditions that are often associated with a tic disorder include anxiety, obsessive-compulsive behaviors, and ADHD.[4] While data suggest that up to 85 percent of persons with chronic motor and vocal tics will have a co-occurring condition, most children develop transient tics that come and go and then stop after a time. While up to 20 percent of children present to their clinician with tics, only about 0.5 percent develop chronic tics that last into adulthood.

Clinical trials are imperfect, and percentiles are sometimes flawed, but the incidence of a substantial co-occurring condition is probably low for most children.

Other cognitive and psychological conditions that can sometimes occur in people with a tic disorder are highlighted in chapter 3. Some children may have speech and language difficulties, challenges with sensory processing, or difficulties with learning. Psychological conditions that have been described in persons with Tourette's disorder include impulse control disorder, disruptive behavior disorder, mood disorder, autism spectrum disorder, self-injurious behaviors, sleep disorder, and various personality disorders. These psychological disorders are generally diagnosed in people who do not have tics. They are generally associated with a co-occurring condition and not with a tic disorder. If concerns arise, the parent should discuss matters with the child's clinician, who might then refer the child for neuropsychological testing or a psychological evaluation.

It is helpful to realize that the core symptoms of a co-occurring condition will likely be present before most children develop tics. Suppose there are no symptoms of anxiety, obsessive-compulsive behaviors, or ADHD when the tics begin. In that case, parents may feel reassured that symptoms of these co-occurring conditions are less likely to arise.

My child has a tic disorder and ADHD. What can be done to help with both of these issues? A tic disorder and ADHD can develop in the same child, but not necessarily at the same time. Generally, the symptoms of ADHD begin much earlier than the tics. Not long ago, clinicians believed that stimulants used for ADHD caused or "unmasked" a tic disorder.[5] This theory is not valid. New clinical trials have shown that stimulants can decrease the frequency of tics.[6] So why did people think that stimulant medication caused the tics? The answer might be uncovered if one considers the typical age of onset of these two disorders. Children with ADHD generally show symptoms in preschool, but teacher comments are often lacking until the child enters kindergarten or first grade. Once the child is within a formal school setting, teacher concerns result in testing. Sometimes a stimulant medication like methylphenidate (Ritalin) is prescribed if the child is diagnosed with ADHD. Whether treated or not, children with ADHD will sometimes develop a tic disorder. The onset of a tic disorder generally occurs after the symptoms of ADHD become clear. Since treatment of ADHD began before the tics developed, the tics were often blamed on the medication.

New evidence from clinical trials has shown that stimulants can reduce tics in children with ADHD.[5,7] It seems that appropriate treatment of ADHD has a beneficial effect on the tic symptoms. These trials show that while stimulants do not cause the tics and can be helpful for most, people treated with stimulants may experience an increase in their tics. The clinician may consider reducing the dose or changing the medication if this occurs.

In place of a stimulant, guanfacine or clonidine might be tried. Guanfacine and clonidine are second-line FDA-approved medications for ADHD, and they can also help to reduce tics.[8] Therefore, if the stimulant is not tolerated, guanfacine or clonidine might help alleviate the symptoms of both conditions when they occur in the same child. These medications are not as good as stimulants for ADHD,[9] so the conditions' relative impact must be considered. For example, if a child has challenges keeping attention and the tics are relatively minor, a stimulant might be used. For a child where tics are the most troublesome problem, guanfacine or clonidine might be used. A third alternative would be to use a stimulant along with guanfacine or clonidine. Methylphenidate and guanfacine[10] or methylphenidate and clonidine are sometimes used together.

Atomoxetine (Strattera) is another good alternative for those with tics, ADHD, and oppositional and aggressive behaviors related to ADHD.[11,12] Atomoxetine is a nonstimulant, norepinephrine reuptake inhibitor. It is FDA approved for ADHD in adults and children.[13] Atomoxetine does not appear to worsen tics, but it may not be as effective as other medications for tics.[14] As with any medications, the potential benefits, potential side effects, risks, and treatment alternatives should be discussed in detail with the child's clinician.

My child has tics and ADHD. Is guanfacine better than clonidine? Guanfacine and clonidine are FDA-approved medications for ADHD, and the medications can be helpful for tics.[8] Guanfacine and clonidine both work by stimulating a specific (alpha-2 adrenergic) receptor in the brain. While clonidine is 10 times more powerful than guanfacine, guanfacine is a more precise medication, as it better targets the appropriate brain receptor. Guanfacine would seem to be the preferred medication for tics and ADHD, as it lasts longer and may have fewer side effects than clonidine.[15,16] However, the American Academy of Neurology gives clonidine moderate confidence for treating tics, while it gives guanfacine a lower score.[17] A nighttime dose of clonidine can help if the child has difficulty falling sleep at bedtime, as a result of either hyperactivity or increased tics in the evening. An increase in tics at bedtime can certainly interfere with sleep. The higher potency of clonidine may help reduce the tics and provide a small amount of sedation that can help with sleep. Ultimately the choice of medication and the time of day at which it is given depend on the individual patient, their symptoms, and the opinion of their clinician.

My child has tics. Do they also have OCD? Obsessive-compulsive behaviors are somewhat common in children with tics. It can be difficult for the clinician to distinguish complex tics from compulsions, as both can result in repetitive movements. However, the repetition of tic-like movements in a series of twos, threes, or more can help to reach a diagnosis of obsessive-compulsive behavior. Children who count their tics are more likely to have OCD than tics, though they might have both. Other non-tic-like obsessive-compulsive behaviors, such as lining up objects and certain rigid routines, are often present. A correct diagnosis is needed, as the treatment options are different. If the child has both tics and obsessive-compulsive movements, a joint approach to treatment may be needed.

Tics and obsessive-compulsive disorder

A 14-year-old girl was referred to a neurologist for evaluation of odd arm and leg movements. She had a prior history of nose-scrunching, lip-puckering, and shoulder-shrugging movements that started when she was 5 years old. These movements had come and gone, but she developed more complex and repetitive stretching movements of her arms and legs that had not changed over five years. When asked, the girl said that she could suppress the movements by concentrating but needed to make these stretching movements or something really bad would happen to her. She needed to stretch three times to feel better, but sometimes she needed to do it more. She was doing well in school and had many friends. When seen in the office, the neurologist noted frequent blinking and occasional stretching movements. She was not aware of the blinking. The rest of her examination was normal. She was sent for a psychological evaluation and received cognitive behavioral therapy for tics and obsessive-compulsive behaviors.

Just because a person has obsessive-compulsive behaviors does not mean that they have OCD. In technical terms, the *Diagnostic and Statistical Manual of Mental Disorders* criteria for OCD specify the presence of compulsions or obsessions that are time-consuming (over one hour per day) or cause distress or functional impairment. Obsessions are characterized by recurrent and persistent thoughts, impulses, or urges that are unwanted and intrusive and cause distress or anxiety.[5] Compulsions are defined as repetitive behaviors or mental acts that the individual feels driven to perform in response to an obsession or rigidly applied rules. The thoughts or behaviors act to prevent or reduce anxiety about a perceived dreaded event or situation.

A child who counts the tic movements may have obsessive-compulsive behaviors. However, there are other differences between OCD and tics. Actions associated with OCD seem to relieve anxiety related to an obsession. In contrast, movements associated with tics alleviate the feeling of a premonitory urge, sometimes described as a physical tension or a sensation. OCD can also occur in persons without tics, but the behaviors seem more related to avoiding contamination or dirt. Obsessive-compulsive symptoms may be present early in childhood, but the symptoms peak later than the onset of tics.[18] Therefore, children who demonstrate tics and obsessive-compulsive-like behaviors need to be monitored so that treatment can be adjusted if required.

My child has obsessive-compulsive behaviors and tics. What treatments are available? The first-line treatment of OCD is cognitive behavioral therapy. Selective serotonin reuptake inhibitors (SSRIs) are helpful for OCD but may not always help to relieve tics.[19] For those with tic-related OCD who do not respond to cognitive behavioral therapy and SSRIs, there is some evidence that antipsychotic medication, such as risperidone and aripiprazole, can improve both tics and obsessive-compulsive behaviors.[20]

Do people with tics also have an intellectual disability? Evidence suggests that children who meet the diagnostic criteria of Tourette's disorder are at risk of associated learning disabilities, executive function difficulties, and other neurodevelopmental problems.[21] This should not imply that children with chronic motor and vocal tic disorder have a disability or will develop learning problems. Indeed, most children presenting with tics in the movement disorder clinic seem to have average or even advanced intellectual ability. As with any child, concerns about an intellectual disability call for a psychoeducational assessment through the school district. These assessments will find both strengths and weaknesses, as discussed in chapter 4. Finding the child's strengths can help the parent and teacher restore confidence in a child who seems to be lagging behind other children in their school class.

How can I find the best clinician? Finding the best clinician to help a child with tics requires careful consideration. The clinician with ability in diagnosing and treating a tic disorder might be a physician, advanced practice provider (APP), advanced practice registered nurse (APRN), or psychologist. First, one should ask, "What kind of specialist is best for my child?" A parent should consider whether the child should see someone specializing in neurological or psychological disorders (see chap. 4). The neurologist would be a good choice for a person with isolated motor tics. A psychologist might be better for a person with tics and one or more co-occurring conditions, such as anxiety, obsessive-compulsive behavior, or ADHD. Sometimes both specialists are needed, and one specialist may send the patient to another for their opinion. A psychiatrist or nurse practitioner (NP) might be needed if the symptoms are severe and the psychologist believes that medications could help. A therapist offers psychological treatments, such as CBIT (see chap. 4). The therapist might collaborate closely with a neurologist, a psychologist, and/or a psychiatrist. This team offers a multidisciplinary approach. The team works closely to supply a treatment plan that will work best for the particular child.

Once the type of specialist is found, the parent or patient should find out who the best clinician in their area might be. It is nice to find someone who is pleasant and can relate to you and your child. Most clinicians in training decide early on whether they like to treat children. The pediatric neurologist receives training in general pediatrics, neurology, and child neurology. A pediatric psychiatrist trains in psychiatry and then completes subspecialty training in child and adolescent psychiatry. A child psychologist generally requires a doctoral degree (PhD or PsyD). Only a few US states allow practicing as a psychologist with a master's degree. The APRN, sometimes called an NP, is a nurse who has met advanced educational and clinical practice requirements. They often supply services in community-based settings but can also practice in specialty care and inpatient hospital units. An APP is an APRN/NP or physician assistant who also has a master's or doctoral degree (note that an APP can also be a nurse midwife or a certified registered nurse anesthetist). After all their years in training, these clinicians are generally well prepared to care for children. The referring health care provider might have experience collaborating with a particular specialist, whom they found to be excellent, and can make a proper referral with someone who has experience evaluating and treating a tic disorder.

Does the age of the clinician matter? People sometimes like to see a young clinician who recently completed training and received up-to-date instruction. Seeing an older clinician also has its advantages. They have more clinical experience and may have treated other children like yours.

If the visit is enjoyable for the child and the clinician listens to and responds to your questions, you might have found the right person. If you think you have found a good clinician, but the treatment is not working, allow the clinician time to find something that works. Not all patients respond to the same medication. It is usual for the clinician to adjust the dose or the time of day the child takes their medication. Occasionally, the medication needs to be changed. In addition, some children show an improvement in tics but then relapse. Let the clinician know when this happens. The child might need a different treatment plan.

How might the clinician follow the effects of treatment? Parents often want to know how long it will take for a particular treatment to start working. This is a difficult question for clinicians to answer. Tics can cycle and change in type, intensity, and frequency. It is generally difficult for the patient to determine whether their tics changed as a result of the natural variations in symptoms or external interventions such as counseling, therapy, or medications. It is unlikely that treatment will produce a complete remission in tics over a short period. Treatments take time, and their positive effects may require weeks or months. Furthermore, a small or moderate symptom improvement is often difficult for the child or their parent to appreciate. Treatments that supply some relief should not be abandoned too quickly. An objective way of following the tic severity is needed. Recording a weekly tic rating score on a calendar can supply a simple but reasonable means of assessing the response to treatment. The score uses a range of 1–10, where 10 is the worst. The score is recorded by the parent—with or without input from the child—every week on a calendar or chart. Rather than relying on memory, the tic score supplies a numerical measure that can objectively determine whether the treatment plan is helpful.

I cannot find a psychologist or a psychiatrist for my child. What can I do? Limited access to mental health care is a challenge that seems to have no end. Persons needing help in rural communities may need to drive miles to be seen by a health care worker. The widespread use of telemedicine has helped this issue. But even those living in major metropolitan areas have challenges obtaining needed health care. Finding a psychologist or psychiatrist can be an overwhelming task. Parents of a nonverbal child or a child with autism spectrum disorder are especially burdened. The waitlist for most, if not all, psychiatry clinics is long, and the wait time to be seen is often many months. The availability of child psychologists and psychiatrists dropped even further owing to the COVID-19 pandemic. Social isolation, fear of becoming infected with the virus, and lack of social interactions were difficult for most people. However, it seemed to have a major effect on school-aged children. These pandemic-related stressors produced a high burden on access to mental health care professionals.

The best approach to finding a psychologist and a psychiatrist may be to find health care professionals who accept the child's health care insurance plan. Next, the parent or patient should consider which of those professionals best suit their child's needs. The parent should also consult with their child's medical team. The pediatrician, neurologist, or social worker might have specific recommendations and may have developed a relationship with certain professionals. The next step is to get on a waitlist. The parent should ask about a waitlist and put themselves on call should there be an opening. Calling the office now and again but not making a fuss or a complaint can make the receptionist aware that the parent is interested in finding a visit sooner. Finally, once the appointment is booked, the parent should cancel any appointments they might have made with another psychologist or psychiatrist. Being late to an appointment will likely reduce the time that the clinician will be able to spend with your child. Not showing up for an appointment wastes time that the clinician could use to help other children.

What should I do if my child will not talk to their therapist? Therapy sessions can help reduce tics and anxiety in children and adolescents. A lighthearted discussion of one's problems and successes can be fun and helpful for a child, especially with someone other than their parents. Opening up to a stranger takes time, and trust needs to develop. The therapist might be terrific and have come highly recommended, but they might not be a good fit for the child. The conversation between the patient and therapist is generally held in private to form trust. If things are not going well, the child may complain that the therapy is making their problems worse, and the therapist might report that the child is not talking to them. Discussion with the child and therapist might help matters. That said, a possible outcome is that the parent will need to search for another therapist who might bond better with their child.

What should I tell my child's teacher? Tics are very common in children, and most schoolteachers will be well acquainted with the disorder. Still, a child with motor and vocal tics can be challenging for the instructor when simultaneously engaging children in a classroom. A child with persistent vocalizations will add to the teacher's already challenging environment. Movements might be noticed by a teacher, but audible tics might be misconstrued as attention-seeking or oppositional behaviors. Children with tics and a co-occurring condition such as ADHD can be a real challenge for the teacher and the other students in class. The parents of other children might hear about the child with tics, which can put additional stress on the child with tics and their family. A parent-teacher discussion before the start of the new school year or in the first weeks of school can prevent misunderstandings that can lead to a stressful learning environment and incorrect disciplinary action against the child.

Parents should also listen very carefully to feedback from their child's teacher. On rare occasions, children with tics may take advantage of the situation. The child should be aware that they are not excused from other abnormal or disruptive classroom behaviors. Parents might also be perplexed when their child's teacher says that they have not seen or heard any tics. Teachers who are occupied with other tasks may not notice the tics. Alternatively, the child may adequately hide or suppress their tics in the classroom. As highlighted in chapter 1, the child who can suppress the tics in school may be more likely to have a tic storm once they return home.

What should I do if my child gets behind in school? By closely watching their child's school grades, the parent shows that they care about the child's education, and the child learns that school performance is important. Variations in school grades are common, as the child may be more interested in one subject than another. A severe decline in the child's grades should raise concerns that something is not quite right. Consulting with the child's teacher is helpful. They may offer insights into a problem that has a solution. Children may not perform well in autumn, when school first begins. This can be a problem if the child is out of school during the summer months. Returning to school, it may take weeks for some children to catch up with the rest of their class. Keeping the child engaged in learning during the summer recess should be considered. A summer learning program planned well in advance may be more acceptable to the child and prevent recurrence of the problem. It will also place the child at a considerable advantage over their classmates when school begins in the fall.

Children who are behind in school and are struggling to keep up with their classmates may experience stress. It will become more challenging for them to catch up with others as time goes on. The pressure will likely worsen the symptoms of co-occurring conditions such as anxiety and increase the frequency and severity of the tics. This may further isolate the child from their classmates. Supplying after-school or summer learning may help reduce stress.

Many children with a tic disorder are exceptionally bright. If the child shows promise but does poorly in school, they could have the inattentive type of ADHD. Alternatively, the parents may have a gifted child who is bored with the subject discussion and is not interested in repeatedly reviewing the same topic. The child does not have the means to voice their frustration, so they sit through the class but occupy their time thinking about other things that are more interesting to them. Rather than supplying added schoolwork, the better approach might be to advance the child into a more intellectually proper learning environment. Skipping a grade or two may be allowed in some school districts, but skipping grades can cause social stress. The intellectually bright child must also show advanced social skills to fit in with older classmates.

How can I speak with my child about their tics? The parents of a child with tics often ask, "What can we say to our child that will help them?" The typical answer is "Don't say anything." According to a study with 126 children aged 9–17 years, the most common tic-provoking interaction was the child being told to stop ticcing (72 percent).[22] This was followed by receiving comfort (59 percent) and being laughed at or teased (35 percent). However, it is a good idea for parents to occasionally discuss the problem with their child. Good communication shows the child that the parent cares about them, and it can help the child cope with stressful situations that the parent might not know about. Certainly, the parent should avoid criticizing the child for their tics. Parents sometimes confront their children when the tics first begin. They are often confused about what is happening to the child. They may also believe that the child is seeking attention. This is particularly common if the child first develops vocal tics. The younger child may be unaware of their tics. When a parent asks the child what they are doing, the child may appear confused. Some older children may laugh and tell the parent that doing the tics makes them feel good. The adolescent might become annoyed with the parent, as the tics will surely increase. It is always proper for parents to talk to their children about their successes and problems. Bringing up the topic when the child is not having tics is counterproductive. The tics will likely resurface. Finding the right time to talk about the tics is essential.

Should I be afraid that my child will be bullied at school? There are many reasons why a parent will bring a child with a tic disorder to see a physician. The parent is often concerned about how their child's friends might interpret the movements and/or sounds. Tics generally start between 4 and 6 years of age. Other children do not seem to notice or comment on the tics when the child is in first, second, or third grade. At this age, children are rapidly developing complex social skills. However, an older student might be excluded from social activities if they do not fit in with the rest of the crowd. Such a child can be the target of bullying. Treatment should begin if the tics impact in-school or out-of-school activities. Treatment should not be started because parents are concerned that other students might harass their child. There are better approaches and remedies for this issue. Shying away from aggressive peers will likely encourage bullying and teasing. Being forthcoming—"I have tics, and what is your problem?"—might be the better approach. Consultation with the school counselor can supply valuable insights and recommendations for each child.

Should I let my child with tics use an electronic tablet? Tablets, smartphones, and computers seem to be the mainstay of communication and learning in schools. The technology gives students new ways to learn different concepts.[23] They allow flexible take-home assignments and new ways to monitor academic performance. Studies have shown that a well-designed digital interactive learning program can support the enhancement of knowledge and thinking skills.[24] However, some digital media can also have harmful effects on behavior and thinking skills.[23,25] Many parents note that their child's tics increase when they are relaxing, watching videos, or playing games on their electronic device. According to one study with 126 children aged 9–17 years, the most common tic-provoking activity was watching television or playing video games (92 percent).[22] This was followed by coming home after school (88 percent), homework (80 percent), the classroom (78 percent), and going to public places (78 percent). It is clear that tics will diminish during periods of goal-directed behavior.[26] However, gaming might provide overstimulation of the visual and auditory sensory system, as well as understimulation once the game has stopped. There may be other reasons as well. The author Mark Twain claimed that "too much of anything is bad." A parent should use their own judgment about how much time is allowed on the electronic device.

Are there any activity limitations for someone with a tic disorder? There is good evidence that routine physical activity or exercise can offer health benefits to a person with a tic disorder.[27] According to the Tourette Association of America, there is no study that proves that a particular form of exercise will reduce tics or improve related symptoms for everybody.[28] In general, there are no known proposed activity limitations for someone with tics. On occasion, a tic might interfere with an activity such as playing baseball. On rare occasions, a complex tic might potentially impair driving. When the safety of the person with a tic disorder, or others, is in jeopardy, the issue should be discussed with the clinician. Some activity restriction may be called for.

I stopped driving

A 16-year-old girl with Tourette's disorder returned to the clinic. Her motor and vocal tics had decreased substantially following several sessions of CBIT. However, she had developed a new complex tic where she would suddenly need to bring both hands up into the air. This happened once when she was practicing driving with a parent. She had stopped driving and was working on a new tic-blocking technique with her therapist.

Should I believe what I hear and read on social media? Parents use social media to access support groups such as the Tourette Association of America. Correspondence with medical therapists or clinicians can be very beneficial. The parent of a child with tics may gain valuable information from other parents or relatives. However, the severity and the duration of a tic disorder differ substantially between people. Further, the response to the treatment of one person with tics might be different from that of another. Therefore, the experience of a family member or an internet acquaintance might be unhelpful. Due to the sheer volume of available material, finding helpful information online is challenging, and the internet is ripe with both knowledge and disinformation. It can be difficult for the parent to know what is real, imaginary, or even a scam. Exceptional one-of-a-kind brain imaging scans that a board-certified radiologist does not review or special blood tests that a certified laboratory does not process may be uninterpretable to other clinicians. "Abnormal" results can lead to expensive and potentially dangerous medications, treatments, or formulations. As such, miracle treatments offered online might be viewed with some skepticism. If nonstandard tests or treatments had proven benefits, they would be discussed in national and international meetings and used routinely by medical professionals eager to improve their patients' lives. Knowledge is valuable, and discussing one's online findings with the child's pediatrician or medical specialist can add more insight.

Humanism for a Child with a Tic Disorder

Humanism is broadly defined as a philosophical stance that emphasizes the individual and social potential of human beings. The Arnold P. Gold Foundation characterizes humanism in health care as a respectful and compassionate relationship between physicians, as well as other members of the health care team, and their patients.[29] Humanism demands that this respectful and compassionate relationship with the patient also extends to their families, friends, and teachers. This section will discuss several potential family and social issues that might develop during the course of a tic disorder.

How do a person's tics affect their family? Tics can be puzzling and annoying to parents and other family members, especially when the tics first begin. It may initially appear that the child is making the movements or sounds on purpose. As such, family members may initially react to the tics in negative ways. They may unknowingly tease the child, and on rare occasions the parents may scold or even discipline their child who has just developed the tics. Such improper, but sometimes understandable, reactions by parents and family members to the movements or vocalizations seem more likely to occur before the child receives a diagnosis of a tic disorder. Unpleasant comments from parents and family members will heighten the child's anxiety and may therefore make the tics worse. Even if the child knows that they have tics, there is little they can do to stop them.

The impact of a chronic tic disorder may be quite challenging for both the patient and their family. Embarrassment is a problem for the school-aged child, whose classmates, as well as their parents, might spread the news through gossip that the child is making odd movements and/or sounds. Persistent and unpleasant tics also risk changing the social behavior of the family. The child's movements and sounds can sometimes become a personal embarrassment for the family, and they may fear that they will lose their social network. Parents may at times become uncomfortable attending family functions where the main topic of conversation could become their child with tics. There is a concern that the family may eventually grow distant from their long-term friends and acquaintances.

Family members and friends who want to help may relate stories of how someone they knew had tics and a particular treatment cured them. The parents may feel pressured to try a specific vitamin or medication, as they heard that it helped someone else's child. Friends may search the internet for specialists and therapists who advertise their cures online. Some people become critical if they think that the parents are not doing enough to help the child.

While the parents' friends and family want to do their best to help, the advice they receive could be better. The pressure to do more for the child with tics can place the family in a challenging and socially stressful position. This pressure, if it occurs, may be a transient issue, as people may tire of the discussion and revert to more typical topics of conversation. Other times, the family may not receive further invitations to social gatherings.

If parents find themselves in such a position, they should remain committed to the diagnosis and treatment plans that they have developed with their child's clinician. It is best to write down family members' concerns and suggestions and discuss these with the child's clinician at a follow-up visit. Suggestions by family and friends can seem helpful, but not all of their ideas are proper.

What about the siblings? The sibling of a person with a tic disorder may also be bothered by the movements and sounds, especially if they share a bedroom. The sibling without tics might also be concerned about social embarrassment. The sibling may be questioned by neighbors or teased by their friends. This places the sibling in an uncomfortable position of choosing between their friends and their brother or sister with tics. This challenging situation could have an impact on them for years to come. A child must try not to socially abandon their brother or sister with tics. Open communication between parents and their children is always necessary. Parents might consider preparing their children for questions from friends and neighbors. One answer might be, "My brother has tics, and he is getting help from his doctor. A lot of us have tics, you know." These issues can become quite complex for the entire family, so discussing such problems with the therapist or clinician can help find a good approach to dealing with them.

How do a person's tics affect their schoolteacher? When a child first develops tics, at the typical age of 4–6 years, they often do not recognize the movements and/or vocalizations. This lack of recognition by the child can be difficult for a teacher to understand. The teacher might ask, "How could he not know that he was making a loud squeak during class?" Or, they might say, "He is trying to cause a disruption!" Purposeful disruptive behavior by a child with a tic disorder is unusual. However, this behavior may occur if the child with tics also has ADHD. The tics can get wound up in the child's hyperactivity, and distinguishing between the two can be very difficult for a teacher with many students. The teacher will benefit from the guidance of the child's diagnosis and a treatment plan. A 504 plan with the student can help the teacher better navigate the situation. Communication between the patient, parent, teacher, and clinician is essential.

How can a family show compassion for the person with tics? While parents and families worry about their child with tics and want to find the best clinician to help them, it is essential to remember that their child might also be very concerned and face challenges at school and home. Talking to the child and asking about their problems and tics is very important. It is not a good idea to talk about the tics too often, as this may increase the tic symptoms, but having an occasional conversation with the child about their tics is a good thing. Leaving the child with tics at home while taking the sibling without tics to a social event has drawbacks. Treating the child with compassion and care will help them feel more secure and may help reduce the disorder's impact on the child.

Hope for the Future

Since Gilles de la Tourette, neurologists, psychologists, psychiatrists, and scientists have spent countless hours thinking about tic disorders. Clinical trials have been performed to see which people are at risk and which treatments might be best. Pathologists have looked into the brain's anatomy to see what, if anything, might be wrong. Geneticists have looked at specific genes to see whether particular changes are shared between persons with tics. All of the data together point to subtle changes that develop within the basal ganglia. Physicians, scientists, and physician-scientists, including those in the Bamford Laboratory at the Yale School of Medicine, have examined the more extensive brain pathways responsible for rational and goal-directed behaviors and those that encode reflexive movements (fig. 5.1).[30] They have also examined the small changes in connections between brain cells that help repetitive movements and behaviors turn into habits. For more information, see https://medicine.yale.edu/lab/bamford/.

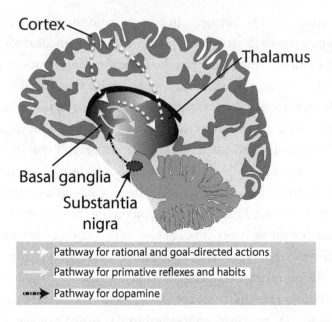

Cortex

Thalamus

Basal ganglia

Substantia nigra

- - -> Pathway for rational and goal-directed actions
——> Pathway for primitive reflexes and habits
■-■-■> Pathway for dopamine

Figure 5.1 Depicted are brain pathways that contribute to the formation of habits. New evidence from the Bamford Laboratory shows that two major brain pathways participate in movements and behaviors. One pathway promotes and maintains habits and allows for primitive reflexes or responses to unexpected sensations. This pathway includes a circuit between the basal ganglia and the thalamus (*white solid lines*). Another pathway allows for rational and goal-directed behaviors. This circuit consists of a loop between the brain's cortex, the basal ganglia, and the thalamus (*white dashed lines*). The loop uses the brain cortex to plan and coordinate movements and behaviors. Both pathways are modified by dopamine (*black dashed line*).

New genetic tools and electrophysiological probes are now used to study normal and abnormal behaviors. These experiments will show more clearly how habits are formed and changed. This challenging and time-consuming research promises to help us understand better how tics occur. Finding specific targets will allow the development of specialized treatments to end the premonitory urge without affecting other brain functions. Without the urge, there is no need for a tic.

Appendix

Resources for Parents, Patients, Clinicians, and Teachers

Information about tics and Tourette's disorder can be found on the Tourette Association of America website at https://tourette.org/. The association describes comprehensive behavioral intervention for tics here: https://tourette.org/research-medical/cbit-overview/.

To assess the symptoms of attention-deficit/hyperactivity in a school-aged child, parents and teachers can download the Vanderbilt Assessment Scales of the National Institute for Children's Health Quality here: https://www.nichq.org/sites/default/files/resource-file/NICHQ-Vanderbilt-Assessment-Scales.pdf.

Patients or their parents who are considering medications for a tic disorder can review a summary of the American Academy of Neurology's practice guideline recommendations at https://n.neurology.org/content/92/19/896.

Seideman and Seideman provide another good review on medications for Tourette's disease, though it is primarily written for clinicians: https://www.ncbi.nlm.nih.gov/pmc/articles/PMC7337131/.

Information on ongoing clinical trials for treating tic disorders and Tourette's disorder is available at https://clinicaltrials.gov/.

Glossary

antipsychotics. Medications that reduce the symptoms of psychosis

anxiety. A feeling of fear, dread, and uneasiness

attention-deficit/hyperactivity disorder (ADHD). Children with ADHD have trouble paying attention and may have difficulty controlling impulses; those with ADHD may also be overactive

basal ganglia. A deep part of the brain that controls learned movements, habits, and behaviors

chorea. A movement characterized by brief, irregular muscle contractions that are not repetitive or rhythmic and appear to flow from one muscle to the next

cognitive behavioral therapy. A psychotherapeutic approach to treating several psychological disorders, such as anxiety disorder and obsessive-compulsive disorder

co-occurring conditions. Disorders like anxiety, obsessive-compulsive disorder, and ADHD that occur more commonly in persons with tics

coprolalia. An offensive complex vocal tic

copropraxia. An involuntary and inappropriate rude gesture

disease. A condition that impairs function and is associated with certain signs and symptoms

dopamine. A neurochemical that helps to program movements and habits

echolalia. Repeating what others say

echomimia. Repeating the mouth movements of others

echopraxia. Repeating what others do

electroencephalogram (EEG). An electrical study that is used to measure brain activity

exposure response prevention therapy. A type of cognitive behavioral therapy that is used to block tics by performing a competing response

habit reversal therapy. A type of cognitive behavioral therapy that is used to block tics by performing a competing response to the premonitory urge

habit tic. A tic that is produced by repeated movements

hysteria. Overwhelming and unmanageable emotional behaviors

institutional review board. A group of experts who review the design of proposed studies and monitor a biomedical research program that involves human subjects

magnetic resonance imaging (MRI). Imaging that uses a large magnet and radio waves to examine brain structure

neuromodulator. A brain chemical that finely tunes the activity of brain cells

neuroplasticity. The ability of brain circuits to change through reorganization

neuropsychology. The study of how the brain affects the way people think and behave

neurotransmitter. A chemical within the brain that allows one brain cell to communicate with another

obsessive-compulsive disorder (OCD). A disorder in which people have recurring unwanted thoughts, ideas, or sensations (obsessions) that make them feel driven to do something repetitively (compulsions)

organic disease. A term that is used to describe a brain problem that might be found on a neurological examination or a particular test

paroxysmal disorder. A disorder characterized by sudden, uncontrollable, and intermittent symptoms

personality trait. A person's characteristic pattern of thoughts, feelings, and behaviors

premonitory urge. A sensation that occurs just before a tic

psychogenic nonepileptic attack. A convulsion that appears to be a seizure but often has atypical features; an EEG is generally normal during the episode

psychosis. A severe mental disorder in which thoughts and emotions are so impaired that contact is lost with external reality

rage attack. An extreme temper tantrum that may be seen with oppositional defiant disorder

receptor. A structure on a brain cell that responds to a neurotransmitter

repurposed medication. A medication designed for one disorder that is used for another

tic storm. Persistent, unrelenting tics that may occur after long periods of tic suppression

transient tics. Tics that last just a few weeks or months

Notes

Chapter 1. Tics and Tourette's Disorder

1. Leckman JF, King RA, Bloch MH. Clinical features of Tourette syndrome and tic disorders. *J Obsessive Compuls Relat Disord*. 2014;3:372–379.

2. Ganos C, Ogrzal T, Schnitzler A, Münchau A. The pathophysiology of echopraxia/echolalia: relevance to Gilles de la Tourette syndrome. *Mov Disord*. 2012;27:1222–1229.

3. Teive HA, Chien HF, Munhoz RP, Barbosa ER. Charcot's contribution to the study of Tourette's syndrome. *Arq Neuropsiquiatr*. 2008;66:918–921.

4. Yorston G, Hindley N. Study of a nervous disorder characterized by motor incoordination with echolalia and coprolalia (the introduction and case studies of Gilles de la Tourette's 1885 paper). *Hist Psychiatry*. 1998;9:97–101.

5. Gilles de la Tourette G. *Étude sur une affection nerveuse caractérisée par de l'incoordination motrice accompagnée d'écholalie et de coprolalie (jumping, latah, and myriachit)*. Paris: Bureaux du Progrès médical; 1885.

6. Charcot J-M. *Leçons du mardi à la Salpêtrière policliniques. Notes de cours de MM Blin, Charcot et Colin*. Paris: Bureaux du Progrès médical; 1887–1888.

7. Gilles de la Tourette G. La maladie des tics convulsifs. *La Semaine Médicale*. 1899;19:153–156.

8. Dowbiggin IR. *Inheriting Madness: Professionalization and Psychiatric Knowledge in Nineteenth-Century France*. Berkeley: University of California Press; 1991.

9. Kushner HI. A brief history of Tourette syndrome. *Brazilian Journal of Psychiatry*. 2000;22:76–79.

10. Fernandez TV, State MW, Pittenger C. Tourette disorder and other tic disorders. In: Geschwind DH, Paulson HL, Klein C, eds. *Handbook of Clinical Neurology*. Amsterdam: Elsevier; 2018:343–354.

11. Hirschtritt ME, Lee PC, Pauls DL, et al. Lifetime prevalence, age of risk, and genetic relationships of comorbid psychiatric disorders in Tourette syndrome. *JAMA Psychiatry*. 2015;72:325–333.

12. Singer HS. Neurobiology of Tourette syndrome. *Neurol Clin.* 1997;15: 357–379.

13. Bamford IJ, Bamford NS. The striatum's role in executing rational and irrational economic behaviors. *Neuroscientist.* 2019;25:475–490.

14. Bamford NS, Wightman RM, Sulzer D. Dopamine's effects on cortico-striatal synapses during reward-based behaviors. *Neuron.* 2018;97:494–510.

15. Costa VD, Tran VL, Turchi J, Averbeck BB. Dopamine modulates novelty seeking behavior during decision making. *Behav Neurosci.* 2014;128: 556–566.

16. Bamford NS, McVicar K. Localising movement disorders in childhood. *Lancet Child Adolesc Health.* 2019;3:917–928.

17. Glimcher PW. Understanding dopamine and reinforcement learning: the dopamine reward prediction error hypothesis. *Proc Natl Acad Sci U S A.* 2011;108 Suppl 3:15647–15654.

18. McKinley JW, Shi Z, Kawikova I, et al. Dopamine deficiency reduces striatal cholinergic interneuron function in models of Parkinson's disease. *Neuron.* 2019;103:1056–1072.

19. Hesse M. What does addiction mean to me. *Mens Sana Monogr.* 2006;4: 104–126.

20. Wang W, Dever D, Lowe J, et al. Regulation of prefrontal excitatory neurotransmission by dopamine in the nucleus accumbens core. *J Physiol.* 2012;590:3743–3769.

21. Wang W, Darvas M, Storey GP, et al. Acetylcholine encodes long-lasting presynaptic plasticity at glutamatergic synapses in the dorsal striatum after repeated amphetamine exposure. *J Neurosci.* 2013;33:10405–10426.

22. Wong MY, Borgkvist A, Choi SJ, Mosharov EV, Bamford NS, Sulzer D. Dopamine-dependent corticostriatal synaptic filtering regulates sensorimotor behavior. *Neuroscience.* 2015;290:594–607.

23. Bamford NS, Zhang H, Joyce JA, et al. Repeated exposure to metham-phetamine causes long-lasting presynaptic corticostriatal depression that is renormalized with drug readministration. *Neuron.* 2008;58:89–103.

24. Bruggeman R, van der Linden C, Buitelaar JK, Gericke GS, Hawkridge SM, Temlett JA. Risperidone versus pimozide in Tourette's disorder: a compara-tive double-blind parallel-group study. *J Clin Psychiatry.* 2001;62:50–56.

25. Dion Y, Annable L, Sandor P, Chouinard G. Risperidone in the treatment of Tourette syndrome: a double-blind, placebo-controlled trial. *J Clin Psychophar-macol.* 2002;22:31–39.

26. Gilbert D. Treatment of children and adolescents with tics and Tourette syndrome. *J Child Neurol.* 2006;21:690–700.

27. Cassano GB, Baldini Rossi N, Pini S. Psychopharmacology of anxiety disorders. *Dialogues Clin Neurosci.* 2002;4:271–285.

28. Kellner M. Drug treatment of obsessive-compulsive disorder. *Dialogues Clin Neurosci.* 2010;12:187–197.

29. Bamford NS, Zhang H, Schmitz Y, et al. Heterosynaptic dopamine neurotransmission selects sets of corticostriatal terminals. *Neuron.* 2004;42:653–663.

30. Bamford NS, Robinson S, Palmiter RD, Joyce JA, Moore C, Meshul CK. Dopamine modulates release from corticostriatal terminals. *J Neurosci.* 2004;24:9541–9552.

Chapter 2. Diagnosing Tics and Tourette's Disorder

1. Kessler RC, Amminger GP, Aguilar-Gaxiola S, Alonso J, Lee S, Ustün TB. Age of onset of mental disorders: a review of recent literature. *Curr Opin Psychiatry.* 2007;20:359–364.

2. Nowogrodzki A. The world's strongest MRI machines are pushing human imaging to new limits. *Nature.* October 31, 2018.

3. Lichtman J, Pfister H, Reid C. Connections in the brain [online]. Accessed May 6, 2024. https://www.rc.fas.harvard.edu/case-studies/connections-in-the-brain/#:~:text=One%20cubic%20millimeter%20of%20cerebral,6%2C000%20synapses%20with%20neighboring%20cells.

4. Ignjatovic V, Lai C, Summerhayes R, et al. Age-related differences in plasma proteins: how plasma proteins change from neonates to adults. *PLOS One.* 2011;6:e17213–e17213.

5. Scahill L, Specht M, Page C. The prevalence of tic disorders and clinical characteristics in children. *J Obsessive Compuls Relat Disord.* 2014;3:394–400.

6. Ganos C, Martino D, Pringsheim T. Tics in the pediatric population: pragmatic management. *Mov Disord Clin Pract.* 2017;4:160–172.

7. Browne HA, Hansen SN, Buxbaum JD, et al. Familial clustering of tic disorders and obsessive-compulsive disorder. *JAMA Psychiatry.* 2015;72:359–366.

8. Leckman JF, King RA, Bloch MH. Clinical features of Tourette syndrome and tic disorders. *J Obsessive Compuls Relat Disord.* 2014;3:372–379.

9. Groth C, Mol Debes N, Rask CU, Lange T, Skov L. Course of Tourette syndrome and comorbidities in a large prospective clinical study. *J Am Acad Child Adolesc Psychiatry.* 2017;56:304–312.

10. Bloch MH, Peterson BS, Scahill L, et al. Adulthood outcome of tic and obsessive-compulsive symptom severity in children with Tourette syndrome. *Arch Pediatr Adolesc Med.* 2006;160:65–69.

11. Pringsheim T, Okun MS, Muller-Vahl K, et al. Practice guideline recommendations summary: treatment of tics in people with Tourette syndrome and chronic tic disorders. *Neurology.* 2019;92:896–906.

12. Scharf JM, Miller LL, Gauvin CA, Alabiso J, Mathews CA, Ben-Shlomo Y. Population prevalence of Tourette syndrome: a systematic review and meta-analysis. *Mov Disord.* 2015;30:221–228.

13. Bloch MH, Leckman JF. Clinical course of Tourette syndrome. *J Psychosom Res.* 2009;67:497–501.

14. Rizzo R, Gulisano M, Cali PV, Curatolo P. Long term clinical course of Tourette syndrome. *Brain Dev.* 2012;34:667–673.

15. Eapen V, Robertson MM. Are there distinct subtypes in Tourette syndrome? Pure-Tourette syndrome versus Tourette syndrome-plus, and simple versus complex tics. *Neuropsychiatr Dis Treat.* 2015;11:1431–1436.

16. Ercan-Sencicek AG, Stillman AA, Ghosh AK, et al. L-histidine decarboxylase and Tourette's syndrome. *N Engl J Med.* 2010;362:1901–1908.

17. Yu D, Sul JH, Tsetsos F, et al. Interrogating the genetic determinants of Tourette's syndrome and other tic disorders through genome-wide association studies. *Am J Psychiatry*. 2019;176:217–227.

Chapter 3. Associated Conditions

1. Hirschtritt ME, Lee PC, Pauls DL, et al. Lifetime prevalence, age of risk, and genetic relationships of comorbid psychiatric disorders in Tourette syndrome. *JAMA Psychiatry*. 2015;72:325–333.

2. Ganos C, Martino D, Pringsheim T. Tics in the pediatric population: pragmatic management. *Mov Disord Clin Pract*. 2017;4:160–172.

3. Tourette's Syndrome Study Group. Treatment of ADHD in children with tics: a randomized controlled trial. *Neurology*. 2002;58:527–536.

4. Mulligan HF, Anderson TJ, Jones RD, Williams MJ, Donaldson IM. Tics and developmental stuttering. *Parkinsonism Relat Disord*. 2003;9:281–289.

5. Pauls DL, Leckman JF, Cohen DJ. Familial relationship between Gilles de la Tourette's syndrome, attention deficit disorder, learning disabilities, speech disorders, and stuttering. *J Am Acad Child Adolesc Psychiatry*. 1993;32:1044–1050.

6. Houghton DC, Capriotti MR, Conelea CA, Woods DW. Sensory phenomena in Tourette syndrome: their role in symptom formation and treatment. *Curr Dev Disord Rep*. 2014;1:245–251.

7. Deak MC, Stickgold R. Sleep and cognition. *Wiley Interdiscip Rev Cogn Sci*. 2010;1:491–500.

8. Fariba KA, Gokarakonda SB. Impulse control disorders [online]. Accessed May 7, 2024. https://www.ncbi.nlm.nih.gov/books/NBK562279/.

9. Frydman I, Mattos P, de Oliveira-Souza R, et al. Self-reported and neurocognitive impulsivity in obsessive-compulsive disorder. *Compr Psychiatry*. 2020;97:152155.

10. Jakuszkowiak-Wojten K, Landowski J, Wiglusz MS, Cubała WJ. Impulsivity in anxiety disorders. A critical review. *Psychiatr Danub*. 2015;27 Suppl 1:S452–455.

11. Porteret R, Bouchez J, Baylé FJ, Varescon I. ADH/D and impulsiveness: prevalence of impulse control disorders and other comorbidities, in 81 adults with attention deficit/hyperactivity disorder (ADH/D). *Encephale*. 2016;42: 130–137.

12. Wright A, Rickards H, Cavanna AE. Impulse-control disorders in Gilles de la Tourette syndrome. *J Neuropsychiatry Clin Neurosci*. 2012;24:16–27.

13. Robertson MM, Cavanna AE, Eapen V. Gilles de la Tourette syndrome and disruptive behavior disorders: prevalence, associations, and explanation of the relationships. *J Neuropsychiatry Clin Neurosci*. 2015;27:33–41.

14. National Institute of Mental Health. Any mood disorder [online]. Accessed May 7, 2024. https://www.nimh.nih.gov/health/statistics/any-mood-disorder.

15. Torres F. What is depression? [online]. Accessed May 7, 2024. https://www.psychiatry.org/patients-families/depression/what-is-depression.

16. National Institute of Mental Health. Major depression [online]. Accessed May 7, 2024. https://www.nimh.nih.gov/health/statistics/major-depression.

17. Robertson MM. Mood disorders and Gilles de la Tourette's syndrome: an update on prevalence, etiology, comorbidity, clinical associations, and implications. *J Psychosom Res.* 2006;61:349–358.

18. National Institute of Mental Health. Bipolar disorder [online]. Accessed May 7, 2024. https://www.nimh.nih.gov/health/topics/bipolar-disorder.

19. Centers for Disease Control and Prevention. What is autism spectrum disorder? [online]. Accessed May 7, 2024. https://www.cdc.gov/ncbddd/autism/facts.html.

20. Canitano R, Vivanti G. Tics and Tourette syndrome in autism spectrum disorders. *Autism.* 2007;11:19–28.

21. Darrow SM, Grados M, Sandor P, et al. Autism spectrum symptoms in a Tourette's disorder sample. *J Am Acad Child Adolesc Psychiatry.* 2017;56:610–617 e611.

22. Mathews CA, Waller J, Glidden D, et al. Self injurious behaviour in Tourette syndrome: correlates with impulsivity and impulse control. *J Neurol Neurosurg Psychiatry.* 2004;75:1149–1155.

23. Fariba KA, Gupta V, Kass E. Personality disorder [online]. Accessed May 7, 2024. https://www.ncbi.nlm.nih.gov/books/NBK556058/.

24. Wilson S, Stroud CB, Durbin CE. Interpersonal dysfunction in personality disorders: a meta-analytic review. *Psychol Bull.* 2017;143:677–734.

25. Ma G, Fan H, Shen C, Wang W. Genetic and neuroimaging features of personality disorders: state of the art. *Neurosci Bull.* 2016;32:286–306.

26. Fortunato A, Tanzilli A, Lingiardi V, Speranza AM. Personality disorders in childhood: validity of the Coolidge Personality and Neuropsychological Inventory for Children (CPNI). *Int J Environ Res Public Health.* 2022;19.

27. Robertson MM, Banerjee S, Hiley PJ, Tannock C. Personality disorder and psychopathology in Tourette's syndrome: a controlled study. *Br J Psychiatry.* 1997;171:283–286.

28. Latas M, Milovanovic S. Personality disorders and anxiety disorders: what is the relationship? *Curr Opin Psychiatry.* 2014;27:57–61.

29. Baer L, Jenike MA. Personality disorders in obsessive compulsive disorder. *Psychiatr Clin North Am.* 1992;15:803–812.

30. Weiner L, Perroud N, Weibel S. Attention deficit hyperactivity disorder and borderline personality disorder in adults: a review of their links and risks. *Neuropsychiatr Dis Treat.* 2019;15:3115–3129.

31. Szuhany KL, Simon NM. Anxiety disorders: a review. *JAMA.* 2022;328: 2431–2445.

32. Weinbrecht A, Schulze L, Boettcher J, Renneberg B. Avoidant personality disorder: a current review. *Curr Psychiatry Rep.* 2016;18:29.

33. Thamby A, Khanna S. The role of personality disorders in obsessive-compulsive disorder. *Indian J Psychiatry.* 2019;61:S114–S118.

34. Brock H, Hany M. Obsessive-compulsive disorder [online]. Accessed May 7, 2024. https://www.ncbi.nlm.nih.gov/books/NBK553162/.

35. Bamford NS, McVicar K. Localising movement disorders in childhood. *Lancet Child Adolesc Health.* 2019;3:917–928.

36. Bonnet C, Roubertie A, Doummar D, Bahi-Buisson N, Cochen de Cock V, Roze E. Developmental and benign movement disorders in childhood. *Mov Disord.* 2010;25:1317–1334.

37. Harris KM, Mahone EM, Singer HS. Nonautistic motor stereotypies: clinical features and longitudinal follow-up. *Pediatr Neurol.* 2008;38:267–272.

38. Singer HS. Motor stereotypies. *Semin Pediatr Neurol.* 2009;16:77–81.

39. Péter Z, Oliphant ME, Fernandez TV. Motor stereotypies: a pathophysiological review. *Front Neurosci.* 2017;11:171.

40. Pringsheim T, Edwards M. Functional movement disorders: five new things. *Neurol Clin Pract.* 2017;7:141–147.

41. Heyman I, Liang H, Hedderly T. COVID-19 related increase in childhood tics and tic-like attacks. *Arch Dis Child.* 2021;106:420.

42. Hull M, Parnes M, Jankovic J. Increased incidence of functional (psychogenic) movement disorders in children and adults amidst the COVID-19 pandemic: a cross-sectional study. *Neurology: Clinical Practice.* 2021:10.1212/CPJ.0000000000001082.

43. Zea Vera A, Bruce A, Garris J, et al. The phenomenology of tics and tic-like behavior in TikTok. *Pediatr Neurol.* 2022;130:14–20.

44. Cavanna AE, Purpura G, Riva A, Nacinovich R, Seri S. Neurodevelopmental versus functional tics: a controlled study. *J Neurol Sci.* 2023;451:120725.

45. Baslet G, Bajestan SN, Aybek S, et al. Evidence-based practice for the clinical assessment of psychogenic nonepileptic seizures: a report from the American Neuropsychiatric Association Committee on Research. *J Neuropsychiatry Clin Neurosci.* 2021;33:27–42.

46. Oto M, Reuber M. Psychogenic non-epileptic seizures: aetiology, diagnosis and management. *Advances in Psychiatric Treatment.* 2018;20:13–22.

47. Smith SJ. EEG in the diagnosis, classification, and management of patients with epilepsy. *J Neurol Neurosurg Psychiatry.* 2005;76 Suppl 2:ii2–7.

48. Chopade TR, Bollu PC. Hemifacial spasm [online]. Accessed May 7, 2024. https://www.ncbi.nlm.nih.gov/books/NBK526108/.

49. Titi-Lartey OA, Patel BC. Benign essential blepharospasm [online]. Accessed May 7, 2024. https://www.ncbi.nlm.nih.gov/books/NBK560833/.

50. Vives-Rodreguez A, Robakis D, Bamford NS. Treatment of neurological symptoms in Wilson disease. In: Schilsky ML, ed. *Management of Wilson Disease.* Totowa, NJ: Humana Press; 2018:107–120.

51. Zimbrean PC, Schilsky ML. Psychiatric aspects of Wilson disease: a review. *Gen Hosp Psychiatry.* 2014;36:53–62.

52. Merical B, Sánchez-Manso JC. Chorea [online]. Accessed May 7, 2024. https://www.ncbi.nlm.nih.gov/books/NBK430923/.

53. Yilmaz S, Mink JW. Treatment of chorea in childhood. *Pediatr Neurol.* 2020;102:10–19.

54. Swedo SE, Leonard HL, Garvey M, et al. Pediatric autoimmune neuropsychiatric disorders associated with streptococcal infections: clinical description of the first 50 cases. *Am J Psychiatry.* 1998;155:264–271.

55. Schrag AE, Martino D, Wang H, et al. Lack of association of group A streptococcal infections and onset of tics: European Multicenter Tics in Children Study. *Neurology.* 2022;98:e1175–e1183.

56. Rhee H, Cameron DJ. Lyme disease and pediatric autoimmune neuro-psychiatric disorders associated with streptococcal infections (PANDAS): an overview. *Int J Gen Med.* 2012;5:163–174.

57. Zibordi F, Zorzi G, Carecchio M, Nardocci N. CANS: childhood acute neuropsychiatric syndromes. *Eur J Paediatr Neurol.* 2018;22:316–320.

58. Tourette Association of America PANDAS/PANS Workgroup. PANDAS/PANS and Tourette syndrome (disorder) [online]. Accessed April 10, 2024. https://tourette.org/research-medical/pandas-pans-and-tourette-syndrome-disorder/.

59. Singer HS, Hong JJ, Yoon DY, Williams PN. Serum autoantibodies do not differentiate PANDAS and Tourette syndrome from controls. *Neurology.* 2005;65: 1701–1707.

60. Singer HS, Gilbert DL, Wolf DS, Mink JW, Kurlan R. Moving from PANDAS to CANS. *J Pediatr.* 2012;160:725–731.

61. Gilbert DL, Mink JW, Singer HS. A pediatric neurology perspective on pediatric autoimmune neuropsychiatric disorder associated with streptococcal infection and pediatric acute-onset neuropsychiatric syndrome. *J Pediatr.* 2018;199:243–251.

62. Andhale R, Shrivastava D. Huntington's disease: a clinical review. *Cureus.* 2022;14:e28484.

63. Cepeda C, Bamford NS, Andre VM, Levine MS. Alterations in corticostriatal synaptic function in Huntington's and Parkinson's diseases. In: Steiner H, Tseng KY, eds. *Basal Ganglia Structure and Function.* San Diego: Elsevier; 2010: 607–623.

Chapter 4. Treatment and Care

1. Singer HS. The treatment of tics. *Curr Neurol Neurosci Rep.* 2001;1: 195–202.

2. Bamford NS, McVicar K. Localising movement disorders in childhood. *Lancet Child Adolesc Health.* 2019;3:917–928.

3. Pringsheim T, Okun MS, Muller-Vahl K, et al. Practice guideline recommendations summary: treatment of tics in people with Tourette syndrome and chronic tic disorders. *Neurology.* 2019;92:896–906.

4. Verdellen C, van de Griendt J, Hartmann A, Murphy T, Group EG. European clinical guidelines for Tourette syndrome and other tic disorders. Part III: behavioural and psychosocial interventions. *Eur Child Adolesc Psychiatry.* 2011;20:197–207.

5. Anderson NP, Feldman JA, Kolko DJ, Pilkonis PA, Lindhiem O. National Norms for the Vanderbilt ADHD Diagnostic Parent Rating Scale in Children. *J Pediatr Psychol.* 2022;47:652–661.

6. Purpura DJ, Lonigan CJ. Conners' Teacher Rating Scale for preschool children: a revised, brief, age-specific measure. *J Clin Child Adolesc Psychol.* 2009;38:263–272.

7. Gomez R, Vance A, Watson S, Stavropoulos V. ROC analyses of relevant Conners 3-Short Forms, CBCL, and TRF scales for screening ADHD and ODD. *Assessment.* 2021;28:73–85.

8. Reynolds CR, Kamphaus RW. *The Clinician's Guide to the Behavior Assessment System for Children.* New York: Guilford; 2002.

9. Kendall PC, Puliafico AC, Barmish AJ, Choudhury MS, Henin A, Treadwell KS. Assessing anxiety with the Child Behavior Checklist and the Teacher Report Form. *J Anxiety Disord.* 2007;21:1004–1015.

10. Hofmann SG, Asnaani A, Vonk IJ, Sawyer AT, Fang A. The efficacy of cognitive behavioral therapy: a review of meta-analyses. *Cognit Ther Res.* 2012;36:427–440.

11. Safren SA, Otto MW, Sprich S, Winett CL, Wilens TE, Biederman J. Cognitive-behavioral therapy for ADHD in medication-treated adults with continued symptoms. *Behav Res Ther.* 2005;43:831–842.

12. Murphy TK, Lewin AB, Storch EA, Stock S, American Academy of Child and Adolescent Psychiatry (AACAP) Committee on Quality Issues (CQI). Practice parameter for the assessment and treatment of children and adolescents with tic disorders. *J Am Acad Child Adolesc Psychiatry.* 2013;52:1341–1359.

13. Ganos C, Martino D, Pringsheim T. Tics in the pediatric population: pragmatic management. *Mov Disord Clin Pract.* 2017;4:160–172.

14. Capriotti MR, Himle MB, Woods DW. Behavioral treatments for Tourette syndrome. *J Obsess-Compuls Rel.* 2014;3:415–420.

15. Duhigg C. Habits: how they form and how to break them. *Fresh Air*, NPR, 2012.

16. Martino D, Pringsheim TM, Cavanna AE, et al. Systematic review of severity scales and screening instruments for tics: critique and recommendations. *Mov Disord.* 2017;32:467–473.

17. Bonnet C, Roubertie A, Doummar D, Bahi-Buisson N, Cochen de Cock V, Roze E. Developmental and benign movement disorders in childhood. *Mov Disord.* 2010;25:1317–1334.

18. Piacentini J, Woods DW, Scahill L, et al. Behavior therapy for children with Tourette disorder: a randomized controlled trial. *JAMA.* 2010;303:1929–1937.

19. McKay D, Sookman D, Neziroglu F, et al. Efficacy of cognitive-behavioral therapy for obsessive-compulsive disorder. *Psychiatry Res.* 2015;225:236–246.

20. Verdellen CW, Keijsers GP, Cath DC, Hoogduin CA. Exposure with response prevention versus habit reversal in Tourettes's syndrome: a controlled study. *Behav Res Ther.* 2004;42:501–511.

21. Rawal A. Google's new health-search engine [online]. Accessed June 21, 2022. https://medium.com/swlh/googles-new-healthcare-data-search-engine-9e6d824b3ccd.

22. Grind K, Schechner S, McMillan R, West J. How Google interferes with its search algorithms and changes your results. *Wall Street Journal*, 2019.

23. Srour M, Lespérance P, Richer F, Chouinard S. Psychopharmacology of tic disorders. *J Can Acad Child Adolesc Psychiatry.* 2008;17:150–159.

24. Jankovic J, Glaze DG, Frost JD, Jr. Effect of tetrabenazine on tics and sleep of Gilles de la Tourette's syndrome. *Neurology.* 1984;34:688–692.

25. Roiz-Santiañez R, Suarez-Pinilla P, Crespo-Facorro B. Brain structural effects of antipsychotic treatment in schizophrenia: a systematic review. *Curr Neuropharmacol.* 2015;13:422–434.

26. Seideman MF, Seideman TA. A review of the current treatment of Tourette syndrome. *J Pediatr Pharmacol Ther.* 2020;25:401–412.

27. Du YS, Li HF, Vance A, et al. Randomized double-blind multicentre placebo-controlled clinical trial of the clonidine adhesive patch for the treatment of tic disorders. *Aust N Z J Psychiatry.* 2008;42:807–813.

28. Song PP, Jiang L, Li XJ, Hong SQ, Li SZ, Hu Y. The efficacy and tolerability of the clonidine transdermal patch in the treatment for children with tic disorders: a prospective, open, single-group, self-controlled study. *Front Neurol.* 2017;8:32.

29. Kuo SH, Jimenez-Shahed J. Topiramate in treatment of Tourette syndrome. *Clin Neuropharmacol.* 2010;33:32–34.

30. Jankovic J, Jimenez-Shahed J, Brown LW. A randomised, double-blind, placebo-controlled study of topiramate in the treatment of Tourette syndrome. *J Neurol Neurosurg Psychiatry.* 2010;81:70–73.

31. Guo H, Ou-Yang Y. [Curative effect and possible mechanisms of topiramate in treatment of Tourette syndrome in rats]. *Zhongguo Dang Dai Er Ke Za Zhi.* 2008;10:509–512.

32. Martínez-Granero MA, García-Pérez A, Montañes F. Levetiracetam as an alternative therapy for Tourette syndrome. *Neuropsychiatr Dis Treat.* 2010;6:309–316.

33. Scahill L, Riddle MA, King RA, et al. Fluoxetine has no marked effect on tic symptoms in patients with Tourette's syndrome: a double-blind placebo-controlled study. *J Child Adolesc Psychopharmacol.* 1997;7:75–85.

34. Marras C, Andrews D, Sime E, Lang AE. Botulinum toxin for simple motor tics: a randomized, double-blind, controlled clinical trial. *Neurology.* 2001;56:605–610.

35. Singer HS, Wendlandt J, Krieger M, Giuliano J. Baclofen treatment in Tourette syndrome: a double-blind, placebo-controlled, crossover trial. *Neurology.* 2001;56:599–604.

36. Bruggeman R, van der Linden C, Buitelaar JK, Gericke GS, Hawkridge SM, Temlett JA. Risperidone versus pimozide in Tourette's disorder: a comparative double-blind parallel-group study. *J Clin Psychiatry.* 2001;62:50–56.

37. Dion Y, Annable L, Sandor P, Chouinard G. Risperidone in the treatment of Tourette syndrome: a double-blind, placebo-controlled trial. *J Clin Psychopharmacol.* 2002;22:31–39.

38. Gilbert D. Treatment of children and adolescents with tics and Tourette syndrome. *J Child Neurol.* 2006;21:690–700.

39. Padala PR, Qadri SF, Madaan V. Aripiprazole for the treatment of Tourette's disorder. *Prim Care Companion J Clin Psychiatry.* 2005;7:296–299.

40. Weisman H, Qureshi IA, Leckman JF, Scahill L, Bloch MH. Systematic review: pharmacological treatment of tic disorders—efficacy of antipsychotic and alpha-2 adrenergic agonist agents. *Neurosci Biobehav Rev.* 2013;37:1162–1171.

41. Hollis C, Pennant M, Cuenca J, et al. Clinical effectiveness and patient perspectives of different treatment strategies for tics in children and adolescents with Tourette syndrome: a systematic review and qualitative analysis. *Health Technol Assess.* 2016;20:1–450, vii–viii.

42. Martinez-Ramirez D, Jimenez-Shahed J, Leckman JF, et al. Efficacy and safety of deep brain stimulation in Tourette syndrome: the International Tourette Syndrome Deep Brain Stimulation Public Database and Registry. *JAMA Neurology*. 2018;75:353–359.

43. Schrock LE, Mink JW, Woods DW, et al. Tourette syndrome deep brain stimulation: a review and updated recommendations. *Mov Disord*. 2015;30:448–471.

44. Tourette Association of America. Medical marijuana research: the cannabis consortium review of the literature [online]. Accessed May 8, 2024. https://tourette.org/research-medical/medical-marijuana-research/.

45. Blessing EM, Steenkamp MM, Manzanares J, Marmar CR. Cannabidiol as a potential treatment for anxiety disorders. *Neurotherapeutics*. 2015;12:825–836.

46. Frolli A, Ricci MC, Cavallaro A, et al. Cognitive development and cannabis use in adolescents. *Behav Sci*. 2021;11:37.

47. Yu J, Ye Y, Liu J, Wang Y, Peng W, Liu Z. Acupuncture for Tourette syndrome: a systematic review. *Evid Based Complement Alternat Med*. 2016;2016:1834646.

48. Bamford IJ, Bamford NS. The striatum's role in executing rational and irrational economic behaviors. *Neuroscientist*. 2019;25:475–490.

49. Bamford NS, Zhang H, Joyce JA, et al. Repeated exposure to methamphetamine causes long-lasting presynaptic corticostriatal depression that is renormalized with drug readministration. *Neuron*. 2008;58:89–103.

50. Wang W, Darvas M, Storey GP, et al. Acetylcholine encodes long-lasting presynaptic plasticity at glutamatergic synapses in the dorsal striatum after repeated amphetamine exposure. *J Neurosci*. 2013;33:10405–10426.

51. Baker LA. The biology of relationships: what behavioral genetics tells us about interactions among family members. *De Paul Law Rev*. 2007;56:837–846.

Chapter 5. Support for the Child at School, Home, and Beyond

1. Tourette Association of America. Individual Education Plans & 504 accommodations [online]. Accessed June 20, 2022. https://tourette.org/resources/overview/tools-for-educators/accommodations-education-rights/iep-504-accommodations/.

2. Office for Civil Rights. Protecting students with disabilities [online]. Accessed June 20, 2022. https://www2.ed.gov/about/offices/list/ocr/504faq.html.

3. Tourette Association of America. Classroom strategies and techniques for students with Tourette syndrome [online]. Accessed June 20, 2022. https://tourette.org/resource/classroom-strategies-techniques-students-tourette-syndrome/.

4. Cravedi E, Deniau E, Giannitelli M, Xavier J, Hartmann A, Cohen D. Tourette syndrome and other neurodevelopmental disorders: a comprehensive review. *Child Adolesc Psychiatry Ment Health*. 2017;11:59.

5. Ganos C, Martino D, Pringsheim T. Tics in the pediatric population: pragmatic management. *Mov Disord Clin Pract*. 2017;4:160–172.

6. Osland ST, Steeves TD, Pringsheim T. Pharmacological treatment for attention deficit hyperactivity disorder (ADHD) in children with comorbid tic disorders. *Cochrane Database Syst Rev.* 2018;6:CD007990.

7. Tourette's Syndrome Study Group. Treatment of ADHD in children with tics: a randomized controlled trial. *Neurology.* 2002;58:527–536.

8. Seideman MF, Seideman TA. A review of the current treatment of Tourette syndrome. *J Pediatr Pharmacol Ther.* 2020;25:401–412.

9. Cortese S, Adamo N, Del Giovane C, et al. Comparative efficacy and tolerability of medications for attention-deficit hyperactivity disorder in children, adolescents, and adults: a systematic review and network meta-analysis. *Lancet Psychiatry.* 2018;5:727–738.

10. McCracken JT, McGough JJ, Loo SK, et al. Combined stimulant and guanfacine administration in attention-deficit/hyperactivity disorder: a controlled, comparative study. *J Am Acad Child Adolesc Psychiatry.* 2016;55:657–666 e651.

11. Gorman DA, Gardner DM, Murphy AL, et al. Canadian guidelines on pharmacotherapy for disruptive and aggressive behaviour in children and adolescents with attention-deficit hyperactivity disorder, oppositional defiant disorder, or conduct disorder. *Can J Psychiatry.* 2015;60:62–76.

12. Ledbetter M. Atomoxetine: a novel treatment for child and adult ADHD. *Neuropsychiatr Dis Treat.* 2006;2:455–466.

13. Fedder D, Patel H, Saadabadi A. Atomoxetine [online]. Accessed May 9, 2024. https://www.ncbi.nlm.nih.gov/books/NBK493234/.

14. Allen AJ, Kurlan RM, Gilbert DL, et al. Atomoxetine treatment in children and adolescents with ADHD and comorbid tic disorders. *Neurology.* 2005;65:1941–1949.

15. Chappell PB, Riddle MA, Scahill L, et al. Guanfacine treatment of comorbid attention-deficit hyperactivity disorder and Tourette's syndrome: preliminary clinical experience. *J Am Acad Child Adolesc Psychiatry.* 1995;34:1140–1146.

16. Scahill L, Chappell PB, Kim YS, et al. A placebo-controlled study of guanfacine in the treatment of children with tic disorders and attention deficit hyperactivity disorder. *Am J Psychiatry.* 2001;158:1067–1074.

17. Pringsheim T, Okun MS, Muller-Vahl K, et al. Practice guideline recommendations summary: treatment of tics in people with Tourette syndrome and chronic tic disorders. *Neurology.* 2019;92:896–906.

18. Bloch MH, Leckman JF. Clinical course of Tourette syndrome. *J Psychosom Res.* 2009;67:497–501.

19. Scahill L, Riddle MA, King RA, et al. Fluoxetine has no marked effect on tic symptoms in patients with Tourette's syndrome: a double-blind placebo-controlled study. *J Child Adolesc Psychopharmacol.* 1997;7:75–85.

20. Masi G, Pfanner C, Brovedani P. Antipsychotic augmentation of selective serotonin reuptake inhibitors in resistant tic-related obsessive-compulsive disorder in children and adolescents: a naturalistic comparative study. *J Psychiatr Res.* 2013;47:1007–1012.

21. Burd L, Freeman RD, Klug MG, Kerbeshian J. Tourette syndrome and learning disabilities. *BMC Pediatr.* 2005;5:34.

22. Himle MB, Capriotti MR, Hayes LP, et al. Variables associated with tic exacerbation in children with chronic tic disorders. *Behav Modif.* 2014;38:163–183.

23. Wetzel N, Kunke D, Widmann A. Tablet PC use directly affects children's perception and attention. *Sci Rep.* 2021;11:21215.

24. Bus AG, Takacs ZK, Kegel CAT. Affordances and limitations of electronic storybooks for young children's emergent literacy. *Developmental Review.* 2015;35:79–97.

25. Bavelier D, Green CS, Han DH, Renshaw PF, Merzenich MM, Gentile DA. Brains on video games. *Nat Rev Neurosci.* 2011;12:763–768.

26. Leckman JF, King RA, Bloch MH. Clinical features of Tourette syndrome and tic disorders. *J Obsessive Compuls Relat Disord.* 2014;3:372–379.

27. Kim DD, Warburton DER, Wu N, Barr AM, Honer WG, Procyshyn RM. Effects of physical activity on the symptoms of Tourette syndrome: a systematic review. *European Psychiatry.* 2020;48:13–19.

28. Tourette Association of America. Exercise, sports and Tourette syndrome [online]. Accessed April 10, 2024. https://tourette.org/resource/exercise-sports-tourette-syndrome/.

29. Gold Foundation. Definition of humanism [online]. Accessed April 10, 2024. https://www.gold-foundation.org/definition-of-humanism/#:~:text=Humanism%20in%20healthcare%20is%20characterized,and%20ethnic%20backgrounds%20of%20others.

30. Bamford IJ, Bamford NS. The striatum's role in executing rational and irrational economic behaviors. *Neuroscientist.* 2019;25:475–490.

Index

Page numbers in *italic* refer to illustrations; those in **bold** refer to tables.

autoimmune diseases, 64, 65
avoidant personality disorder, 50

baclofen, **83**, 86
Bamford Laboratory at the Yale School of
    Medicine, 118
basal ganglia: antibodies and, 64; defini-
    tion of, 121; function of, 12–13, 31,
    32, 90, *117*, 118; stimulation of, 87
Behavior Assessment System of Children,
    73
Benadryl (diphenhydramine), 42, **83**,
    86–87
benign paroxysmal torticollis, **53**
benign sleep myoclonus, 52, **53**, 54
Biden, Joe, 35
biofeedback, 72
bipolar disorder, 46
blepharospasm, 62
blinking movement: CBIT treatment of,
    77; MRI scan and, 20; OCD and,
    103; replaced by other symptoms,
    23; self-awareness of, 25; tics and, **18**,
    19, 25, 40, 51, 52, 58, 61; Tourette's
    disorder and, 22
Borrelia burgdorferi, 65
brain, 7, 31, *32*
brain cells, 13, *14*, 15, 20
brain circuits, 7, 8, *14*, 90–91, *117*
brain tumors, 7

cannabidiol (CBD), 87–88
Carroll, Lewis, 35
Catapres (clonidine), **83**
Centers for Disease Control and Preven-
    tion, 47
cerebellum, *32*
Charcot, Jean-Martin, 4, 5, 6, 63
Child Behavior Checklist / Teacher
    Report Form, 73
childhood acute neuropsychiatric
    symptoms (CANS), 65

children with tic disorders: academic
    progress of, 109–10; with ADHD,
    109; bullying of, 111–12; challenges
    of maintaining attention, 96;
    challenges of managing sensory
    input, 98; co-occurring condition,
    116–17; embarrassment of, 115;
    families of, 117–18; humanism for,
    114–15; individualized educational
    plan for, 93–95, 117; interactions
    with siblings, 116; language deficits,
    97–98; limitations of activities for,
    112–13; schoolteachers and, 109,
    116–17; social isolation of, 110, 116;
    special accommodations for, 92–99,
    109; therapies outside the school,
    99; use of electronic devices, 112
chorea, 5, 11, 63, 121
chronic tic disorder, 10, 17, **18**, 37, 46, 48,
    99, 115
clinical trials, 80, 81–82, 100
clonidine, 42, **83**, 84–85, 101, 102
cognitive behavioral therapy (CBT),
    49, 56–57, 70–71, 74, 90, 103,
    121
comorbid disorder, 28
complex motor stereotypies, 52, **53**,
    54–56
comprehensive behavioral intervention
    for tics (CBIT): application of, 71;
    description of, 74–75; length of, 76;
    objectives of, 76; practices of, 75;
    usefulness of, 76–78
compulsions, 104
conduct disorder, 43, 44–45
Conners scale, 73
convulsions, 57, 59, 60
convulsive tic disease, 5–6
co-occurring conditions: chances of
    having, 30–31, 100; common
    problems associated with, 34–42;
    diagnostic of, 33; discovery of, 59;

for students with, 92, 95–96; complex motor stereotypies and, 56; as co-occurring condition, 21, 28, 29, 99; diagnostic of, 103–4; evaluation of, 72, 73; *vs.* impulse control disorder, 43; learning abilities and, 38; medications for, 87–88, 104; sensory intolerance and, 37; sleep problems and, 41; symptoms of, 103, 122; tics and, 67, 102–3; treatment of, 78, 103, 104
obsessive-compulsive personality disorder, 50
oppositional defiant disorder, 43, 44, 45
Orap (pimozide), 83
orbitofrontal cortex, 32
organic disease, 122

paroxysmal disorder, 60, 86, 122
paroxysmal tonic upgaze, 53
pathological studies, 7
pediatric acute-onset neuropsychiatric syndrome (PANS), 65
pediatric autoimmune neuropsychiatric disorders associated with streptococcal infections (PANDAS), 64–65
pediatricians, 66
pediatric psychiatrists, 105–6
personality disorder, 42, 49–50, 51, 100
personality traits, 11, 47, 50, 123
phonic tics, 2
physicians, 105
pimozide, 83, 84, 86
Pitié-Salpêtrière Hospital, 4
placebo effect, 80–81
pneumonia, 65
post-traumatic stress disorder, 59
post-viral encephalitis, 18
premonitory urge: abnormal sensory function and, 37; anxiety and, 28, 72; CBIT for recognition of, 74, 75, 76,

78; definition of, 1, 123; functional movement disorder and, 58; symptoms of, 33; tics and, 8–9, 9, 10, 27, 58, 104
provisional tic disorder, 3–4, 18
psychiatrists, 66, 67, 108
psychoeducational evaluation, 40, 74, 75, 105
psychogenic nonepileptic attack, 59, 60, 123
psychologists, 66, 67, 68, 106, 108
psychosis, 6, 123
psychotherapy, 72
pyromania, 43

rage attack, 45–46, 123
receptors, 11, 14, 15–16, 20, 83, 86, 91, 102, 123
Rehabilitation Act, 93
relaxation exercises, 42, 45, 71–72, 75
repurposed medication, 84, 123
restless legs syndrome, 41
Risperdal (risperidone), 83
risperidone, 83, 86, 104
Ritalin (methylphenidate), 101

Sandifer syndrome, 53
schizophrenia, 6
school counselors, 73–74
seizure: diagnostic of, 54, 62; functional movement disorders and, 57, 59; medications for, 85; symptoms of, 52, 65; tics and, 18, 19, 60–61
selective serotonin reuptake inhibitors (SSRIs), 16, 86, 104
self-awareness, 25
self-injurious behaviors, 49, 58, 100
self-monitoring, 72
sensory processing disorder, 34, 36, 37, 98–99, 100
serotonin, 15, 16

shoulder shrugging: anxiety and, 30; OCD and, 103; replaced with other symptoms, 23; tic disorders and, 3, **18**, 103; Tourette's disorder and, **18**, 22, 51

shuddering attacks, **53**

sleeping disorders, 35, 40, 41–42, 54, 100, 102

sleep-related rhythmic movements, 52, **53**

sniffing, 19, 23, 51

social media: children and, 41, 42, 58, 59, 71; medical information on, 72, 113–14

Social Responsiveness Scale, 48

social workers, 59, 67, 70–71, 73–74, 93, 108

spasmus nutans, **53**

speech disorders, 34, 35–36, 97–98, 100

squinting movements, 25

stereotypies, 54–55, 56

stimulant medications, 16, 101

Strattera (atomoxetine), 101

Streptococcus, 63, 64

stress, 57, 71–72

stretching movements, 103

stroke, 7

stuttering, 35–36

substantia nigra, *32, 117*

supplements, 89

Sydenham's chorea, 63, 64, 65

synapse, 13

teachers, 69, 109, 116

telemedicine, 107

temper tantrums, 45–46

Tenex (guanfacine), **83**

tetrabenazine, **83**

thalamus, *32, 117*

therapists, 66, 67, 105

throat clearing, **18**, 22, 30, 44

tic disorder: age factor, 1, 3, 8, 11, **18**, 22; causes of, 6–8, 10–12, 13, 63–64;

clinical trials, 80–82; co-occurring conditions, 30, 31, 42, 72, 99–101; cues and, 8–9; definition of, 1, 17; disappearance of, 23, 27; disruptive behavior disorders and, 44–45; early descriptions of, 4, 5; family history and, 24–25; genetic explanation of, 7, 10, 11; guidance for parents and teachers, 99–103; *vs.* habits, 10, 13; harm from, 24; impact on child's life, 92, 107, 111, 114–15; internet resources on, 78–79, 113–14, 119; learning abilities and, 21, 104–5, 109–10; mild and transient, 3; psychiatric explanation of, 6–7, 11; *vs.* seizures, 60–61; self-awareness of, 2–3, 25–26; self-taught behavioral therapy, 26–27; sensory intolerance and, 37; sleep deprivation and, 40; statistics of, 21, 22–24; *vs.* stereotypies, 54–55; studies of, 4–6, 10, 118; suppression of, 27; symptoms of, 2, 6, 17, **18**, 26–27, 37, 40; *vs.* Tourette's disorder, 21–22; types of, 1–2; urges and, 8–9, 9, 10; *See also* diagnosis of tic disorder; medications for tic treatment; treatment of tic disorder

tic storm, 9, 86–87, 109, 123

Topamax (topiramate), **83**

topiramate, **83**, 85–86

Tourette, Gilles de la, 4, 5, 6

Tourette Association of America, 82, 94, 113

Tourette's disorder: cognitive abilities and, 34–35; *vs.* convulsive tic disease, 6; co-occurring conditions, 30–31; deep brain stimulation and, 87; diagnostic of, 17, **18**, 19, 21–22, 51–52, 58; family history and, 24–25; *vs.* impulse control disorder, 43; medications for, 22; personality disorders and, 50; statistics of, 21, 24; symptoms of,

About the Author

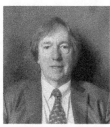

Nigel S. Bamford, MD, is an associate professor in pediatrics, neurology, and cellular and molecular physiology at Yale University. He studied electrical engineering and attended medical school at the University of Utah. After completing a residency in general pediatrics at Columbia-Presbyterian Medical Center in New York, Dr. Bamford received subspecialty training in child neurology at the Neurological Institute of New York and Columbia University. As a physician-scientist specializing in movement disorders, he received a professorship at Columbia University before moving to Seattle to set up the Bamford Movement Disorders Laboratory at Seattle Children's Hospital and the University of Washington. After spending 13 years in Seattle, he moved to Connecticut in 2015, where he cares for children with neurological disorders at Yale New Haven Hospital.

Dr. Bamford specializes in the evaluation and treatment of children with movement disorders. As a physician-scientist funded by the National Institutes of Health, he runs a laboratory investigating the underlying causes of neurological diseases that produce abnormal movements and behaviors. His laboratory uses unique optical techniques, electrophysiology, and behavioral experiments to figure out how circuits that lie deep within the brain can produce motor learning. Learned motor movements include basic activities such as crawling, walking, and running, along with more complex activities such as writing, riding a bike, and driving a car. The brain circuits that encode these movements are called the basal ganglia. The Bamford Laboratory discovered that brain circuits in the basal ganglia change as an animal learns a series of activities to develop a particular skill. These changes in brain circuity, called neuroplasticity, are often helpful since the learned skill may be repeated without needing to think through each step. Unfortunately, neuroplasticity is not all good. The Bamford Laboratory showed that neuroplasticity in basal ganglia circuits could promote addiction to drugs often abused. Neuroplasticity also promotes abnormal movements in Parkinson's disease and Huntington's disease. By examining the brain mechanisms that underlie a tic disorder, investigators can determine what medications and treatments can help those in need.

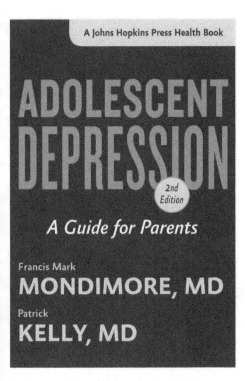
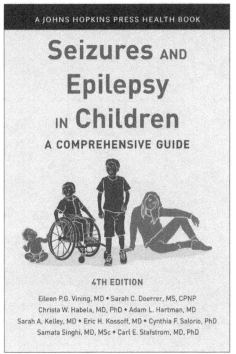